The Power of Bach Flower Remedies for Children

Natural Bach Flower Remedies for Babies, Toddlers, Children and Adolescents

Noah Goldhirsh

Translated from the Hebrew by Noël Canin

BOOKS

Hammersmith Health Books
London, UK

First published in Hebrew in 2022
First published in English in 2023 by Hammersmith Health Books
– an imprint of Hammersmith Books Limited
4/4A Bloomsbury Square, London WC1A 2RP, UK
www.hammersmithbooks.co.uk

Disclaimer: This book was written and illustrated by Noah Goldhirsh. The
methods of diagnosis, adaptation of Bach Flower Remedies and and their uses
to support young people all represent the writer's views and suggestions based
on her knowledge and long-term experience. This book in no way constitutes
a medical or therapeutic prescription nor can it replace conventional therapies.
When necessary, a qualified physician and therapist who specializes in Bach
Flower Remedies and treatment should be consulted for an accurate diagnosis and treatment plan. Under the heading 'A personal experience' this book
includes a variety of illustrative case histories. The personal details of babies,
children and adolescents have been changed in order to protect the privacy of
the individual, and the personal experiences described here have no direct bear-
ing on any baby, child or adolescent whatsoever.

British Library Cataloguing in Publication Data: A CIP record of this book is avail-
able from the British Library.

Print ISBN 978-1-78161-248-4
Ebook ISBN 978-1-78161-249-1

Commissioning editor: Georgina Bentliff
Translated from the Hebrew by: Noël Canin
Typeset by: Julie Bennett of Bespoke Publishing, UK
Cover design by: Madeline Meckiffe
Cover image by: Helen Chapman
Index: Dr Laurence Errington
Production: Deborah Wehner of Moatvale Press Ltd
Printed and bound by: TJ Books Limited, UK

Praise for *The Power of Bach Flower Remedies*

'This book offers a comprehensive and practical guide for utilizing Bach flower remedies in therapy with children. It has proven immensely valuable to me in my work with children and, even as an adult, I have found its insights applicable to my own personal growth.'
Alexandra Madorski, Certified Bach Flowers therapist and children's physical activity coach

'In many situations and challenges that my children encountered over the years, the healing power of Bach Flower Remedies gently influenced them to follow new emotional paths and deal better with their lives. Noah Goldhirsh's important book is a key to understanding the wonderful world of Bach Flower Remedies and accompanies me and my family every day in a practical and useful way.'
Maya Moss, therapist using horse riding

'An accessible and convenient book, which contains all the information I need for taking care of children. It is always there to assist me in preparing extracts for my children and for my patients.'
Lena Madorsky, Certified Bach Flowers therapist, Psychiatric Hospital Nurse and mother of three

'I wholeheartedly recommend Noah Goldhirsh's book, which has helped me take care of myself and of others by using the healing powers of Bach Flower Remedies. You can easily learn and apply the methods in the book, and take care of your child in a natural way.'
Tehila Katya Lubamirski, Certified Bach Flowers Therapist, Body and Mind Treatments

This book is dedicated with enormous gratitude and infinite love to all the Light Entities.
To Mother Earth who always provides us with physical and mental cures.
To my loving husband.
To my children and grandchildren.
May we always live in harmony, love and joy.

Contents

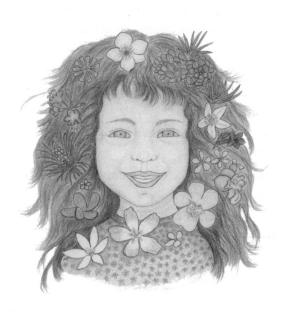

The birth of a book

Nature around us provides remedies for body and mind, balancing and empowering us mentally and physically. Throughout my decades of work as a Holistic Therapist, I have come to realize that the connection to nature and the use of natural remedies can materially help us improve our lives.

I first encountered Dr Bach's flower remedies over 30 years ago and discovered that treatment via these remedies is soothing and supports physical and mental recovery, affecting humans and animals alike in the most remarkable ways.

The use of the enormous healing properties inherent in simple flowers helps us to balance and improve our lives physically and mentally. The flower remedies can be used as treatments in themselves, or as supplements for other healing methods.

I've treated and taught thousands of people how to treat themselves, their children and their pets with Bach Flower Remedies. Infants, children and adolescents tend to respond quickly to these remedies and, having specialized over the years in the treatment of children in varying circumstances, I'm glad to share my knowledge of these unique methods in order to help children of all ages.

Bach Flower Remedies are suitable for any life situation and have proved particularly effective as a supplementary treatment for children and adolescents who suffer from problems such as: fear and anxiety, attention-deficit disorder (ADHD), eating disorders and social difficulties stemming from the Covid-19 epidemic, etc.

Bach Flower Remedies are sold all over the world and are considered a supplement, *not* medication. They can be purchased in the relevant stores and used simply and quickly.

This book offers simple, practical methods for all to use and shows how to enjoy all the inherent healing possibilities of these remedies to improve our health and enable us to lead good, happy and balanced lives.

Introduction

What are Bach Flower Remedies?

Bach Flower Remedies consist of 38 flower remedies created by Dr Edward Bach, a British doctor who lived in England between the years 1886 and 1936, and who specialized in medicine, bacteriology and homeopathy. Dr Bach studied the human mind and ways of healing physical and mental illnesses. In 1930, he discovered and created a new method of treatment, using energetic remedies from flowers for the purpose of achieving balance and physical and mental wellbeing. His most famous compound, created to address acute problems and trauma, is called Rescue Remedy. Bach Flower Remedies are considered a food supplement and sold over the counter, without the need for a prescription in all countries. They are considered a gentle, safe remedy for people and animals of any age.

Dr Bach believed that body and mind were connected and that physical and mental illness derived from oppressive emotions, internal conflict or unresolved life issues. His basic assumption was that the human body was full of life energy and was striving to heal; when the appropriate flower remedies were administered, the body was able to achieve emotional balance and heal itself physically and mentally. He suggested looking for the person's mental conflict and then administering the Bach Flower Remedy that would best treat these conflicts, thus helping that person overcome their difficulties, boosting and balancing their life energy, which would help them recover.

After Dr Bach's death, his followers established a world Bach Flower Remedy Centre at his home, Mount Vernon, in Oxfordsire, UK.

The method of producing Bach Flower Remedies is based on transferring the energy of the flower to water. At the end of the process, brandy is added to preserve the remedy over time.

Over the years, many have claimed that the technique of transferring energy to water is not scientific. However, in 1994, Dr Masaru Emoto began to photograph and document his research regarding experiments with water under varying circumstances. His scientific and orderly research proved that any energy transferred to water transforms this water into another medium, a process that can actually be documented. It is possible to read about his work on the miraculous powers of water and see his extraordinary photographs of the transformation taking place in water. In Dr Masaru Emoto's book, *The Hidden Messages in Water*, published in Japan in 1999, his research shows practical evidence of the extraordinary ability of water to remember and preserve the energy to which it is exposed, enabling us to understand the real and practical foundation of treatment based on Bach Flower Remedies.

Dr Bach paved a new way for understanding and healing human beings by using a simple, particularly active supplement and, in the course of the years during which I have used this method to help people, I have seen how Bach Flower Remedies powerfully affect clients, improving and enriching their lives.

Bach Flower Remedies can be bought in pharmacies and health food stores as a complete kit containing 38 vials of remedies and two bottles of Rescue Remedy. Individual vials can also be purchased as required.

I will end with the words of an adolescent who came to me in the course of his treatment for drug addiction: 'If I'd known there was something so simple and cheap that could calm my body and soul, I wouldn't have wasted so much money on the drugs that have destroyed me and my life...'

Bach Flower Remedies for body and mind

Since the dawn of history, the great spiritual teachers have taught us that we inhabit a vast and infinite universe and that our soul in fact constitutes timeless, infinite, concentrated energy. Each time we choose to come into the world, our soul chooses to live inside a particular physical body and, when our physical body is spent, our soul returns to the energy of the infinite. Each life cycle of the soul within a particular body is known as an 'incarnation', and each human being experiences various incarnations, during which they learn the life lessons required for their spiritual development. In the body of every baby, child or adolescent lives an eternal, spiritual soul that has come into the world to learn physical and mental lessons in the course of life's journey. Children frequently encounter problems in their lives; it is hard for them to find an appropriate balance between body and mind and, in situations of imbalance, they could suffer from internal and external conflict, as well as various illnesses.

An illness is primarily the result of internal conflict and, when a child suffers, Bach Flower Remedies can help the mind to relax and the physical body to gather strength. We can help children at any stage in life by preparing Bach Flower formulas for them. This book provides a great deal of knowledge about the properties of Bach Flower Remedies and the ways in which therapeutic formulas are prepared and best used to help children of any age. Bach Flower Remedies enable us to help our children simply and pleasantly. When the choice of Remedy is accurate, body and mind relax and regain their balance. Bach Flower Remedies are not harmful and so if you have chosen one that doesn't accurately suit the child or adolescent, don't worry. A remedy that isn't accurate will simply have no effect.

Supporting children of all ages with Bach Flower Remedies

The 38 Bach Flower Remedies are meant to address a range of problems, including anxiety, jealousy and outbursts of rage. Each Remedy is meant to address the child or adolescent's characteristic emotional and behavioral problems as detailed in this book. Bach Flower Remedies can help children of all ages and this approach is based first and foremost on profound observation of the child or adolescent's behavior and on listening to what they and their parents say. If the child doesn't yet speak, it is crucial to pay attention to his or her behavior and to listen to what the parents and caregivers say. We can give the child or adolescent a combination of Remedies designed to resolve an acute, short-term problem or, support them in the long term with the help of a Remedy formula meant specifically for them. A deep knowledge of the child or adolescent and an understanding of their situation, wishes and needs is the basis for creating an accurate Bach Flower formula.

The best way to prepare a formula for deep and meaningful support is to use a combination of the three kinds of Remedy, which I describe later:

a Type Remedy (see page 138)
a Situation Remedy (see page 139)
a Support Remedy (see page 140).

Each child or adolescent might need several Remedies of each kind as the human personality is complex and consists of unlimited emotions and behaviors. When we address typical/habitual behavior with Bach

Flower Remedies, we are addressing the consistent behavior pattern of the child or adolescent. When we add Remedies to the formula to address a temporary situation, we are helping the child/adolescent to cope with current difficulties; when we add a Support Remedy to the formula, we are supporting the process of change and helping the child or adolescent to cope with all the things that are bothering them, thus helping them to regain balance and recover mentally and physically. We can occasionally change the composition of the formula in accordance with the changing needs of the child or adolescent, but it is advisable to continue to use a formula that they like and that has helped them, in order to achieve the best possible long-term results.

Since the duration of Bach Flower Remedy use is not limited, it's possible to continue this support for a long period of time, or to return to it every time the child or adolescent needs this help.

Helping children with Bach Flower Remedies for urgent or temporary conditions

Children and adolescents constantly experience processes of change and growth and it is very important to address any temporary problem that appears as soon as possible, to prevent it from becoming a chronic condition. We address a temporary problem with the appropriate Bach Flower Remedies, to which we add Rescue Remedy plus the child or adolescent's Type Remedy.

In various emergency situations, it is advisable to put 4-6 drops of Rescue Remedy in the child or adolescent's mouth, or 6 drops of Rescue Remedy in a glass of water to be sipped slowly.

You can prepare a therapeutic Rescue Remedy spray or a therapeutic cream in advance, based on Rescue Remedy (see instructions on page xx), to be used externally in emergency situations.

In cases where a child or adolescent is already using Bach Flower Remedies and has a personal formula, it is possible in an emergency to give them Rescue Remedy together with their personal formula.

The three-step technique for practical success with Bach Flower Remedies

This technique brings together information regarding the process of using Bach Flower Remedies, detailing the best way to achieve practical, therapeutic success.

The first step: Diagnosis

An accurate diagnosis is the foundation of any successful use of the Remedies. Make time for a diagnostic conversation with the child or adolescent, sit with them and listen deeply to what they say in order to understand their way of thinking, difficulties and wishes.

You can ask them to make a list of their difficulties and the things that are bothering them, then using this as a basis for the diagnostic conversation. Pay attention to their physical and verbal reactions; tell them they can say anything they want to; you are there *with* and *for* them. It isn't necessary to respond verbally to everything they say or to their facial or bodily expressions. Simply listen to them, asking for clarification when necessary in order to understand the situation.

Accurate diagnosis depends on real listening without judgment. Take all the time they need; sit quietly with them, and listen.

When diagnosing babies or very young children who are difficult to talk to, discuss the problem with parents or caregivers in order to understand the issues bothering them and act in accordance with what they tell you about the baby or child's behavior.

Diagnostic stages

1. Ask the child or adolescent what is bothering them and write down their responses in an orderly way. Avoid expressing an opinion.
2. Ask the child or adolescent what they want in their life and write down their responses in an orderly way. Avoid expressing an opinion.
3. If you need clarification on a certain issue, ask your question simply and directly and write down the child's responses in an orderly way. Avoid expressing an opinion.
4. In conclusion, read the main points you have noted to the child or adolescent and ask them if they think what you have written is accurate and true; then make any corrections necessary.
5. Thank the child or adolescent for an honest, sincere conversation and for agreeing to share their innermost feelings.
6. *Only if you are the child or adolescent's parent*, offer them a close, physical gesture like a hug – naturally, *only if they want it.*

The second step: Preparation

It is advisable to prepare the bottle of Bach Flower Remedy somewhere quiet, without external disturbance. If you wish to be completely focused on the preparation process, prepare the bottle on your own and then give the bottle to the child or adolescent. If you wish and are able to share the preparation process with the child or adolescent, ask them if they wish to be present while you prepare it, or whether they'd prefer to receive the prepared bottle. Listen to their response and act according to the child or adolescent's wishes.

Preparation stages

1. Read out the list of what the child or adolescent said and note down next to each problem the name of the flower that best fits this problem.
2. Select a formula that contains up to seven Bach Flower Remedies as detailed on page 138.
3. Write down the formula you have chosen in two places:
    A. Prepare a card for the child or adolescent and note their

> name, date of the diagnosis, and the formula you have cho-
> sen.
> B. On a sticker prepared in advance, note down the selected
>   formula, the name of the child or adolescent and the prepa-
>   ration date of the bottle.
> 4. Prepare a Bach Flower Remedy bottle as detailed on page xxx.

The third step: Using the Remedies

Bach Flower Remedy use is continued for as long as the child or adolescent has mental or physical need of this help. Some children/adolescents
respond quickly, while others do so more slowly. Each child or adolescent has their own pace and we must respect this and support them
through the process.

Treatment stages

1. Give the Bach Flower Remedy you have prepared to the child
    or adolescent and ask them to put 4-6 drops of the remedy in
    their mouth. (NB: When treating small children, parents put the
    required amount into their mouth.)
2. Explain to the child or adolescent that they must take 4-6 drops
    from the bottle at least four times daily and, in addition, they
    can take 4-6 drops from the bottle whenever they feel the need.
3. When necessary, add 4-6 drops from the Bach Flower Remedy
    bottle to the child or adolescent's personal water bottle, as de-
    tailed on page 142.
4. Pay attention to the way the Bach Flower Remedy is taken, the
    right dosage, and consistent doses of the appropriate Remedy
    for as long as is needed.
5. Parents, when you administer Bach Flower Remedies to babies
    or young children, make sure to give them the Remedy formula
    at least four times a day:
    •   first, when the baby or child wakes up in the morning
    •   second, towards noon
    •   third, in the afternoon
    •   fourth, before going to sleep at night
    •   and, in addition, whenever necessary.
6. When the Bach Flower Remedy bottle is almost finished, have

another conversation with the child or adolescent to find out the current situation. It is usually advisable to continue the same formula with the next bottle, but occasionally it is necessary to change one of the formula components. It takes time for children and adolescents to part from problems and old habits. *Remember that each body has its own pace and don't rush to change a winning formula.* The Sages said: 'Never change a winning horse half way up the hill.'

7. If a child or adolescent feels their condition has improved and says they have no further need of the Bach Flower Remedy, sit down with them for another diagnostic conversation. If you see and sense that their condition has improved and the problems have been satisfactorily resolved, you can stop using the Remedies.

8. Remind the child or adolescent and yourself that the Remedies can always be resumed; it is always possible to take Bach Flower Remedies when necessary.

Getting to know the wonder of the Bach Flower Remedies

The pages that follow this will give you an in-depth knowledge of the remarkable Bach Flower Remedies and their extraordinary beneficial effects on young people of all ages. In order to make this book really useful, each Remedy is described in three ways:

1. The first section describes for whom the Remedy is suitable, detailing the conditions in which children and adolescents can profit from its use.
2. The second section describes the effect of the Remedy.
3. The third section presents a 'personal experience', describing a situation in which a child or adolescent is effectively treated with a Remedy. The personal experience is based on real case histories, the personal details of which have been changed to protect individuals' privacy. Each 'personal experience' includes the formula(s) that I adapted to specific situations in the lives of these individuals. When necessary, you can use these formulas as a *basis* for formulas you may wish to create yourself. Carry out as accurate a diagnosis as you can for the child or adolescent and adapt the formula to their personal needs.

After making up the formulas, they can be used in Bach Flower Remedy bottles, sprays and therapeutic creams, as described further on in this book (pages 143-147).

1.
AGRIMONY

Agrimony eupatoria

FOR INNER SADNESS HIDDEN BEHIND
A CHEERFUL FACE

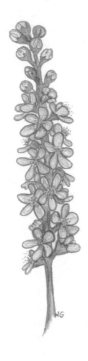

The Agrimony Remedy can help children and adolescents who appear smiling and cheerful but whose external cheerfulness hides sadness, pain, a lack of self-esteem and, sometimes, depression. They occasionally assume the 'face of a happy clown', attempting to amuse people around them and make them laugh, but behind the happy mask hides a sad child or adolescent who avoids telling people about their suffering because they don't want to 'burden' others with their troubles. Such children rely on very few people; it is hard for them to ask for help; and only someone whom they really trust will ever know their inner world. A child or adolescent who needs the Agrimony Remedy tends to avoid arguments, preferring peace at all costs, even if this is only a superficial and external peace.

Agrimony Remedy suits children or adolescents who devote time and effort to making a good impression on friends, parents and teachers. They tend to make light of their suffering, appear carefree and hide their problems when distressed, happily starting afresh with a smile. They tend to suffer from insomnia and, occasionally, from sleep-walking ('moon-sickness'). They are frequently restless and seek excitement.

Adolescents who require the Agrimony Remedy tend to suffer from hidden anxiety and might have suicidal tendencies. They may also use alcohol or drugs to calm down and open up to people.

Warning: In the event of any suicidal tendency, consult a qualified doctor.

Agrimony Remedy helps children and adolescents who suffer from various forms of physical and emotional pain, hiding these by: over-eating, endless viewing of videos on their mobile phones, computer games that go on for hours, viewing and engaging in social networks, drinking alcohol, using drugs, etc.

Agrimony Remedy also helps with allergies, stings, infections and rashes.

Taking the Remedy

Taking Agrimony Remedy provides inner quiet, helping children and adolescents to love themselves, to be able to share their thoughts and actions with others, and to use their humor and courage to express themselves and be free and happy.

Important note: When Agrimony is used as a Type Remedy (page 138), it is advisable to be careful when taking it as part of a first treatment. Agrimony helps children and adolescents to speak their thoughts freely aloud. A child who is used to hiding their true thoughts might be alarmed by this, and people around them might be surprised by their uncharacteristic behavior and respond in a way that could hurt the child. When a child or adolescent grows accustomed to using Bach Flower Remedies and the process is more comprehensible to them, their ability to cope with emotional exposure improves, and the use of Agrimony becomes a more conscious, effective and meaningful process.

A personal experience

Jonathan, aged 3 years, went to a city kindergarten for the first time. When his mother came to fetch him, he gazed at her as if he couldn't believe his eyes, ran into her arms and hugged her for a long time. The kindergarten teacher told her that he had been calm and quiet all day, and Jonathan looked at her silently and smiled.

When his mother asked him, 'How was kindergarten?' he gazed at her in silence. Jonathan continued his silence for several hours and when his mother realized that her happy, talkative little boy had completely stopped talking, she brought him to me.

I prepared a bottle of Bach Flower Remedies for Jonathan with the following formula:

- **Agrimony** – to help him speak and share what had happened in kindergarten with his mother.
- **Rescue Remedy** – for calm and general balance.
- **Star of Bethlehem** – to address the trauma he'd experienced in kindergarten.
- **Walnut** – to improve his ability to transition from one state to another.
- **Mimulus** – to alleviate the tangible fear he'd experienced in kindergarten.
- **Aspen** – to address his unconscious fears.
- **Larch** – to reinforce his self-confidence.

Jonathan took the bottle of Bach Flower Remedies in both hands, held it to his heart, and drank from it again and again. After a few minutes, he gave a huge sigh, turned to his mother and told her: 'Mama, I was so afraid... It was hard for me in kindergarten, I missed you and I cried, and the kindergarten teacher told me that if I went on crying, you wouldn't come to fetch me... I was sad and it was hard for me to stop crying, but I was afraid that if I cried you'd never come, and the kindergarten teacher told me not to tell you, so I stopped talking...'

His mother held him tightly, told him she loved him and that he could always tell her anything. Jonathan was then homeschooled, growing and developing confidently and joyfully.

2.
ASPEN

Populus tremula

FOR FEAR OF THE UNKNOWN

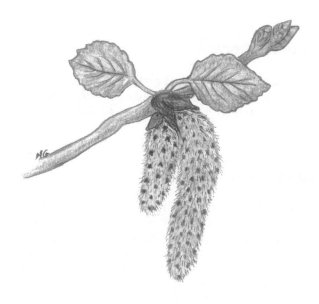

Aspen Remedy helps babies, children and adolescents who suffer from fears and anxieties of an unknown origin. A child in need of Aspen might suffer from recurring nightmares; they might be afraid of certain places; or of imaginary creatures under the bed, etc. They might request a night-light or come into their parents' bed in the middle of the night.

Aspen Remedy is suitable for very sensitive children and adolescents who tend to feel they are unusual, imagine possible disasters, are constantly worried about unknown things, and frequently suffer from sleep problems, such as: trouble falling asleep; frightening dreams; or even sleep-walking ('moon sickness').

Aspen Remedy helps children and adolescents who suffer from extreme sweating, stomach pain, unexplained pain and problems with the urinary tract, such as: incontinence and nocturnal bed-wetting.

It also helps with panic attacks, terror and trembling, and we combine it with many formulas to address different kinds of fear, including for children who have been sexually abused.

Taking the Remedy

Taking Aspen Remedy gives children and adolescents the strength to face their fears openly and confidently, while trusting in their abilities. It helps them to calm down, feel safe and protected, and let go of various fears.

A personal experience

Rachel, a single parent, brought Guy, her 7-year-old son, to me for help. He was afraid to go to the toilet alone or move from one room to another in their home, asking her to go everywhere with him. When I talked to Guy, it turned out that his friends had shown him videos on a mobile phone in which scary creatures jumped out from hidden corners. Consequently, he was afraid that the creatures he'd seen on the mobile phone would lie in wait for him in any dark corner. Once we understood the origin of the problem, I prepared a bottle of Bach Flower Remedies for Guy with the following formula:

- 🌸 **Aspen** – to address his fears of hidden creatures.
- 🌸 **Walnut** – to improve his ability to move from one situation to another.
- 🌸 **Mimulus** – to address his fear of entering the toilet and other rooms on his own.
- 🌸 **Rescue Remedy** – for calm and general balance.
- 🌸 **Star of Bethlehem** – to address the trauma that resulted from viewing the scary videos.
- 🌸 **Larch** – to reinforce his self-confidence.

Guy cheerfully tasted the Bach Flower Remedy combination and liked the flavour. His mother told me that change came swiftly and within two weeks his fears had completely vanished.

3.
BEECH

Fagus sylvatica

FOR ARGUMENTATIVENESS, INTOLERANCE
AND BEING OVERLY CRITICAL

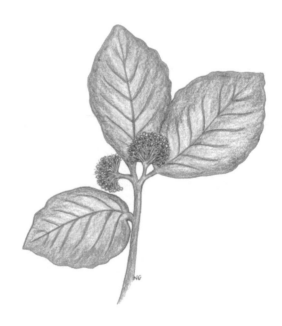

Beech Remedy helps children and adolescents who tend to be critical, impatient, controlling and conceited. A child or adolescent in need of Beech Remedy has difficulty accepting unusual people and situations and will comment on any mistake or flaw they see without considering the feelings of others. A child might behave like this if they feel they aren't sufficiently appreciated or supported; if they feel their parents prefer their siblings; or from a desire to emulate a dominant adult in their life.

Beech Remedy is suitable for helping children who tend to be physically and emotionally tense and rigid, and children and adolescents who enjoy arguing, proving they are right at any cost and controlling the way in which others act. During puberty, Beech Remedy can help adolescents who are full of disappointment and anger, who judge others and who tend to argue with the whole world because they think they know better than anyone else.

Beech Remedy also helps with back and neck pain, or any rigid, tense parts of the body, constipation, hemorrhaging and blocked sensory organs.

Taking the Remedy

Taking Beech Remedy helps children and adolescents to see the beauty of the world around them and enjoy it uncritically, filling their hearts with empathy and tolerance, enabling them to see others' good qualities and abilities, understand their difficulties and know that everyone chooses to cope with life in their own unique way.

A personal experience

A well-known lawyer came to me with his 10-year-old son, Benjamin. He told me that the boy was very tense, had difficulty making friends, suffered from constipation and tended to argue about everything. When I talked to Benjamin, he told me in fluent and witty language that his class mates were childish, useless and stupid, and he didn't have a single 'real' friend. As we talked, he pointed at my bookcase, saying that the shelves were dusty; he said I should clean them. His father, who was sitting next to him, nodded, smiled and said: 'He will make an excellent lawyer; he knows how to argue every issue, show people where they are wrong and tell them what they should do.'

Benjamin smiled proudly, saying: 'Yes, I know how to talk just like my father! But when I tell children in my class what they should do, they just get mad and fight with me, or walk off. Such idiots....'

I prepared a bottle of Bach Flower Remedies for Benjamin with the following formula:

- **Beech** – to calm his tendency to argue.
- **Vine** – to moderate his need to control and tell everyone what to do.
- **Rescue Remedy** – for calm and general balance.
- **Walnut** – to improve his ability to transition from one situation to another.
- **Crab Apple** – to address his constipation.
- **Impatiens** – to alleviate his tension, feelings of pressure and the tendency to quarrel.
- **Water Violet** – to improve his ability to connect with other children.

Benjamin gladly agreed to use the Bach Flower Remedies and, two months later, he was calmer, his constipation had vanished, he was less argumentative, and he had made friends with several children his own age.

4.
CENTAURY

Centaurium umbellatum

FOR THE INABILITY TO SAY 'NO' TO OTHERS

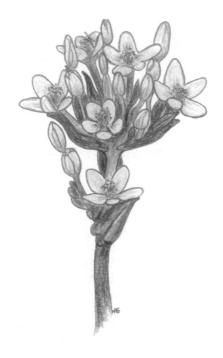

Centaury Remedy can help a quiet, sensitive child who has trouble saying 'no' when asked to do something they don't want to do, because they feel they can't refuse others' demands. Children who need Centaury Remedy try to please their parents, friends and teachers, to help and serve them, and tend to suppress their own needs in order to 'keep the peace' and gain the approval of those around them. They tend to feel tired from the effort of satisfying the needs of others, but don't complain, because they have accustomed themselves to working hard for others. They are likely to become servants for dominant people or the victims of bullies they encounter.

An adolescent who needs Centaury Remedy might be easily influenced by others and join a cult, get addicted to drugs, etc.

Centaury Remedy is suitable for bolstering the child or adolescent's will during an illness, for reinforcement after a tough illness, and for treating addictions.

Taking the Remedy

Taking Centaury Remedy:
- helps children and adolescents to reinforce their self-esteem
- balances their desire to serve and help
- helps them to pay attention to their personal needs, saying 'no' without guilt, and
- helps them to avoid being bound by the wishes of others.

A personal experience

Fourteen-year-old Naomi came to me for help, suffering from physical and mental exhaustion and deterioration in her school work. Her parents told me she was a nice, pleasant, polite girl who took care of her younger siblings, helped her mother with the housework, and even helped the neighbors when necessary. Naomi told me that in addition to the help she gave her parents at home, she helped an elderly neighbor do her shopping, and occasionally helped another neighbor with her children.

'It's hard for me to say "no" when Mama needs my help, and I certainly can't say "no" when our elderly neighbor asks me to go shopping for her, or when our young neighbor tells me she urgently needs my help… I know they all need my help and I'm not complaining, but I'm really tired, and I'm afraid that because I don't have time to study, I won't get good grades in the exams…'

We talked about the importance of self-awareness and the need to be able to say "no" when we feel we can't carry out a certain task, and I prepared a bottle of Bach Flower Remedies for Naomi with the following formula:

- **Centaury** – to balance her desire to help and serve others.
- **Rescue Remedy** – for calm and general balance.
- **Olive** – for mental and physical reinforcement.
- **Walnut** – to improve her ability to transition from one situation to another.
- **Mimulus** – to alleviate her fears of not getting good grades.
- **Cerato** – to reinforce her faith in her inner voice and decisions.
- **Red Chestnut** – to soothe excessive concern for people close to her heart.

After Naomi had used the Bach Flower Remedies for a time, there was a marked improvement in her condition. She began to pay more attention to her inner voice and, today, she makes sure to devote time to her personal needs, not being too quick to put her desires aside because of the requests, needs and demands of others.

5.
CERATO

Ceratostigma willmottiana

FOR INDECISIVENESS AND OVER-DEPENDENCE ON THE OPINIONS OF OTHERS

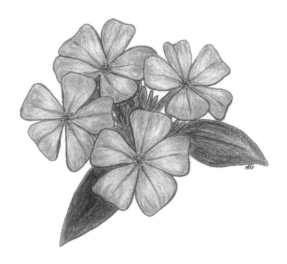

Cerato Remedy can help children and adolescents who have difficulty choosing and being decisive in many areas of their life because of a lack of confidence together with frustration and uncertainty. They tend to ask the opinion of family members or friends about issues that pre-occupy them and act in accordance with their advice, always trying to get outside approval for their actions and choices, not trusting their own judgment or ability to make the right decisions.

A child who needs Cerato Remedy is easily overwhelmed by the opinions of others, asks their friends to be on their side, and tends to be swayed by dominant children. They tend to imitate the behavior, style of address and clothing of the dominant child in the kindergarten or class. During adolescence, their condition might deteriorate and they may be drawn into a bad crowd and negative actions while influenced by others.

A child or adolescent might need Cerato Remedy in situations that require them to make a decision; if they are at an important crossroads in their life; they are also likely to suffer from illnesses that are difficult to diagnose. A combination of Cerato Remedy, Walnut, and Type Remedies (see page 138) unique to their personality in a treatment formula taken over time could help them find their true voice and free themselves from being controlled by others.

Taking the Remedy

Taking Cerato Remedy reinforces the child or adolescent's belief in him/herself, their path, and their decisions, encouraging them to learn to trust their inner voice, distinguish between good and bad and choose inde-pendently, acting in the best way possible.

A personal experience

Sixteen-year-old Dana told me she had difficulty choosing and buying clothes because she couldn't decide what suited her. When she went shopping with her mother, she would go from one store to the other, endlessly trying on clothes and asking her mother a thousand times what she thought of each garment.

One day, she bought a lovely yellow bathing suit she really liked, and invited a friend over to see it. The friend looked at it with critical eyes and said: 'A red bathing suit would have been better.'

Dana told me: 'I immediately ran to my mother and told her we had to go back to the store and exchange the bathing suit. My mother looked at me in despair, saying: "But you liked the yellow bathing suit; why do you want to exchange something just because your friend said so?" At that moment, I realized that my opinion mattered. I tend to ask too many people about things in my life, and I'm influenced by their opinion. It's a real problem; it's impossible to be constantly dependent on the opinions and thoughts of others...'

I prepared a bottle of Bach Flower Remedies for Dana with the following formula:

- **Cerato** – to reinforce her belief in herself, her inner voice and her decisions.
- **Rescue Remedy** – for calm and general balance.
- **Larch** – to reinforce her self-confidence.
- **Walnut** – to improve her ability to transition from one situation to another.
- **Mimulus** – to alleviate her fear of making a mistake or a wrong decision.
- **Aspen** – to address her hidden fears.

Dana used the Bach Flower formula for some time and, a few months later, she told me her life had completely changed. Today she easily makes her own decisions regarding things that matter to her and is even able to advise others.

6.
CHERRY PLUM

Prunus cerasifera

FOR ANGER, OUTBURSTS OF RAGE, AND VIOLENCE

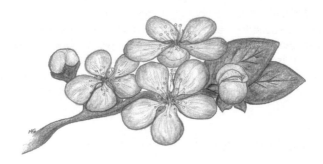

Cherry Plum Remedy helps children and adolescents who suffer from uncontrollable anger and outbursts of violence and hysteria. These outbursts usually appear during periods of emotional and/or physical change, such as: moving house, the birth of a sibling, their parents' divorce, while following an extreme diet, following a period of depression, fear, anxiety, or some profound life upheaval, when they cannot cope with what they are experiencing and they erupt like a volcano. When intense emotions appear, the child or adolescent is afraid of going mad, losing control and doing terrible things. They might be destructive or suicidal or have a strong urge to self-harm or harm others.

Children in need of Cherry Plum Remedy suffer from uncontrollable outbursts of rage; they scream and cry with fury, throw themselves on the floor or hit their head against the wall.

Outbursts of rage might intensify during puberty and many adolescents channel their anger by adorning their bodies with multiple earrings, tattoos, etc. Cherry Plum Remedy addresses outbursts of anger and situations where a child loses control over body functions. It is crucial to combine the Remedy with Walnut and Type Remedies (see page 138) that are unique to the child or adolescent's personality.

As a result of the lockdowns and social isolation during Covid-19, throughout 2020 and 2022, outbursts of rage radically increased among children and adolescents; verbal violence on social networks intensified as well as phenomena of physical and verbal violence in kindergartens and schools. It is advisable to deal with any situation of verbal and/or physical violence immediately to prevent deterioration and, in emergencies, use Rescue Remedy, which includes Cherry Plum Remedy.

Taking the Remedy

Cherry Plum Remedy facilitates emotional balance in the child or adolescent, enabling them to cope courageously, calmly and in a balanced way with the world; it clarifies the young person's thoughts and calms their painful emotions, teaching them to let go of their rage and allow things to pass.

A personal experience

Fifteen-year-old Sun's parents asked me to help him urgently after he was suspended from school for shouting at a teacher and throwing a chair at him. They told me he behaved violently and angrily at home, refusing to listen to them, even going to a tattoo artist without their permission to have a black panther tattooed on his back.

Sun agreed to come to me for help and after a few sessions confided that he felt angry and irritable all the time; a single word could set him off and he was afraid he might go mad. He told me: 'It all started when my parents began fighting all the time and shouting at each other. On one hand, I was glad they got divorced, because it was horrible living with them during the period of their marriage break down. On the other hand, I feel I don't have a real family now; I go from one house to the other, can't rely on them, and my sister is the only one who understands me... I feel I don't have any control over my life, and I tend to lose control in difficult situations, getting upset and shouting just like my parents so they'll see me and notice that I exist... That's why I had a black panther tattooed on my back; it represents strength, control and power for me.'

I prepared a bottle of Bach Flower Remedies for Sun with the following formula:

- **Cherry Plum** – to address his anger and violent outbursts.
- **Rescue Remedy** – for calm and general balance.
- **Walnut** – to improve his ability to move from one house to another and one situation to another.
- **Water Violet** – to alleviate his sense of loneliness and lack of belonging.
- **Star of Bethlehem** – to address the trauma of his parents' divorce.
- **Honeysuckle** – to cope with his past memories.
- **Aspen** – to calm his hidden fears.

Sun tasted a few drops of the formular I prepared for him and said it tasted really good. He continued to take it consistently and, within a few months, his behavior had improved considerably both at home and at school. I saw him again a few years later and he told me that the Bach Flower Remedy had changed his life for the better, helping him to recognize his inner strength, control himself, and deal successfully with life's tests.

7.
CHESTNUT BUD

Aesculus hippocastanum

FOR LEARNING DISABILITIES AND DIFFICULTY LEARNING
FROM PAST EXPERIENCE

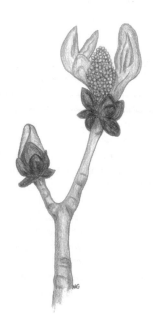

Chestnut Bud Remedy helps children and adolescents with learning difficulties and children who tend to learn slowly and with difficulty, forget things they have already learned, and repeat past mistakes or behavioral patterns that aren't in their best interests.

A child or adolescent in need of Chestnut Bud Remedy quickly learns and excels at a subject that they love, like sport or computer games, but if they have to learn difficult things or things that don't interest them, they learn very slowly, have difficulty focusing and tend to forget things like their satchel or pencil case again and again, despite many reminders.

Chestnut Bud Remedy is effective for difficulties with physical and mental development, as well as for problems with memory and for being stuck and unable to progress in life. Chestnut Bud Remedy is the main essence for helping children and adolescents who suffer from attention-deficit disorder (ADD or ADHD), and it helps treat 'tics' (involuntary movements or sounds) of various kinds.

During the 2020-2022 Covid-19 pandemic, most children and adolescents in the world were separated from their friends, studying via the computer screen. This resulted in deterioration for many children and adolescents who had difficulty learning this way. It is advisable to add Chestnut Bud Remedy to the personal formula of children and adolescents who have difficulty learning, until their studies improve.

Taking the Remedy

Chestnut Bud Remedy helps concentration and focus in the present moment. It also reinforces learning ability and internalization. It helps children and adolescents to learn, to accumulate knowledge and wisdom from their studies and experiences, and to stop repeating past mistakes so they can progress in life.

A personal experience

Ten-year-old Dan was diagnosed with a learning disability and transferred to a special class at school, but his academic situation didn't improve; he sat daydreaming in class, was unable to learn to read or write and constantly postponed doing his lessons both at school and at home.

I prepared a bottle of Bach Flower Remedies for Dan with the following formula:

- **Chestnut Bud** – to improve his ability to concentrate and learn.
- **Rescue Remedy** – for calm and general balance.
- **Walnut** – to improve his ability to transition from one situation to another.
- **Clematis** – to address his tendency to daydream while studying.
- **Larch** – to reinforce his self-confidence.
- **Hornbeam** – for his tendency to procraste.
- **Mimulus** – for fears that stemmed from his failure in school.

I advised Dan to take the formula four times daily and add it to his personal water bottle. Every time Dan then had difficulty in school, he'd take a sip of water with the Bach Flower Remedy and feel better. His parents told me that within a few weeks there was significant improvement in his behavior and learning capability. Today, Dan reads and writes fluently and succeeds in his studies. He loves his Bach Flower Remedy formula and continues to take it on a daily basis.

8.
CHICORY
Cichorium intybus

FOR POSSESSIVENESS AND SELF-PITY

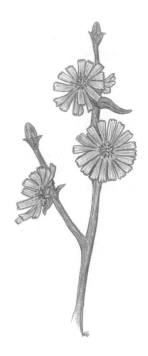

Chicory Remedy can help children and adolescents who have a tendency to try to control and be possessive of people and objects. Children and adolescents in need of Chicory Remedy are in desperate need of love and recognition, usually suffering from a lack of these and the feeling that they aren't loved enough. They will love certain people and publicly, occasionally melodramatically, take care of them, but will always feel they don't receive enough love in return. They are often overwhelmed by emotions and fear of losing those dear to them; they require an abundance of love and a sense of security. A child who needs Chicory Remedy demands a great deal of attention, tends to cry easily and has difficulty being alone.

When in difficulties, they are filled with self-pity and use emotional blackmail to achieve what they want, sometimes even creating an imaginary illness to gain attention.

They are profoundly hurt when they feel they don't receive the respect they deserve, and they might often perceive gifts and money as a declaration of love, emotionally manipulating those close to them in order to receive gifts, and refusing to share their belongings with siblings or friends.

Taking the Remedy

Taking Chicory Remedy reinforces a child or adolescent's confidence and self-esteem, fosters their ability to give with all their heart without demanding anything in return, soothes financial concerns and teaches them how to share with others.

A personal experience

Two-year-old Leo had difficulty being away from his mother or parting from her; he held onto her hand or her clothing. At social encounters with his peers, he refused to share his games or toys with other children, and if someone tried to take one of his toys, he'd immediately burst into tears.

His mother approached me for help and, after discussing his behavior and habits, I prepared a bottle of Bach Flower Remedies for Leo with the following formula:

- **Chicory** – to reinforce his sense of confidence and improve his ability to share belongings.
- **Rescue Remedy** – for calm and general balance.
- **Walnut** – to improve his ability to transition from one situation to another.
- **Larch** – to reinforce his self-confidence.
- **Mimulus** – to treat his fear of being distanced from his mother.
- **Aspen** – to address his hidden fears.

After taking the Bach Flower Remedies for several days, Leo's behavior significantly improved and his mother told me that he had calmed down, was more independent, and was now able to play happily with other children and share his toys with them.

9.
CLEMATIS

Clematis vitalba

FOR 'SPACINESS' AND DAY-DREAMING

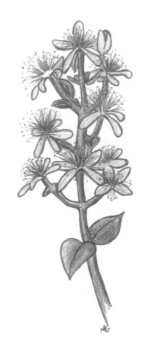

Clematis Remedy helps a child or adolescent who tends to be indifferent to their surroundings, to dream and fantasize, preferring to live in their imagination rather than cope with everyday life. These young people are sensitive, spiritual and impractical, don't pay a lot of attention to what is happening in the present and might forget most of what is said to them. They very much enjoy sleeping and sinking into the world of their dreams, occasionally being able to sleep for many hours.

Children and adolescents in need of Clematis Remedy tend to be pale and sleepy, their eyes stare and their face has a dreamy expression. They aren't attentive to their surroundings and appear to 'drift', sometimes sinking into painting or writing poetry or stories. They tend to bump into objects they don't notice and will sometimes suffer from a poor body image.

Clematis Remedy is suitable for children and adolescents who suffer from difficulty focusing and concentrating; it also addresses states of disconnection and mental confusion resulting from shock due to a physical or mental crisis.

Taking the Remedy

Taking Clematis Remedy can increase the child or adolescent's ability to focus, to take an interest in things, to be aware and practical, and to live in the present and fulfill their life's purpose.

A personal experience

Ten-year-old Lee's teacher told her parents that their daughter was very smart but spent most of her lessons daydreaming and not paying attention to what was happening in the classroom, which was why she wasn't succeeding at her studies.

When I met Lee, I realized that she was mature for her age, smart, pleasant and had a highly developed imagination and a wonderfully complex inner world. She told me that she was afraid of failing her classes but, when the material taught in class didn't interest her, she simply sank into dreams, disassociating from her external environment.

I prepared a bottle of Bach Flower Remedies for her with the following formula:

- **Clematis** – to calm her tendency to daydream at school.
- **White Chestnut** – to calm her thoughts and improve her learning ability.
- **Rescue Remedy** – for calm and general balance.
- **Walnut** – to improve her ability to transition from a dreaming state to one of attention to what was happening in class.
- **Larch** – to reinforce her self-confidence.
- **Mimulus** – to alleviate her fear of failing her classes.

Lee tasted the formula and said, pleased, 'It tastes like chocolate!'

After taking it for some time, her ability to listen and concentrate in class improved; her grades greatly improved; and her teachers were delighted with her success. Lee is very happy with the improvement in her life and continues to take the Bach Flower Remedies when needed, before important exams, etc.

10.
CRAB APPLE

Malus pumila

FOR FEELINGS OF DISGUST AND EATING DISORDERS

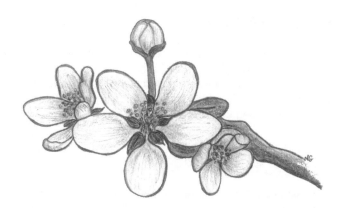

Crab Apple Remedy can help children and adolescents who are disgusted by parts of their body, their environment or other people, and feel a need for excessive cleansing. This Remedy can help a highly sensitive child or adolescent who is disgusted by such things as insects, bodily secretions, eating from someone else's plate and dirt of any kind, and girls who are disgusted by their menstrual cycle and suffer as a result.

Crab Apple Remedy is effective for children and adolescents who tend to get caught up in small things, paying attention to tiny details without seeing the big picture; who suffer from remorse because of something they did in the past and are ashamed of; or who suffer from an eating disorder or obsessive compulsive disorder (OCD).

Crab Apple Remedy is part of the basic formula in the preparation of sprays and creams for various skin problems; it is suitable for external use for skin ailments, and helps children and adolescents who suffer from acne or skin disease.

Taking the Remedy

Crab Apple Remedy successfully helps a variety of skin problems, scratches, cuts or stings.

Taking this Remedy can help children and adolescents relieve the disgust they feel for various things, see things in proportion and calmly accept things that used to stress them in the past.

A personal experience

Seventeen-year-old Sarah suffered from anorexia and was referred to me for supplementary help by her psychologist. Treating patients with eating disorders tends to be long and arduous and it is crucial to be in constant contact with professionals in this field.

Sarah told me that she was disgusted by herself and her image in the mirror, and the thought of eating frightened and disgusted her. She told me very openly that when she ate, she felt as if she was putting something unclean into her body and had to throw it up. Her condition made her avoid others and she was very lonely and disconnected from the world.

I prepared a bottle of Bach Flower Remedies for Sarah with the following formula:

- **Crab Apple** – to alleviate her sense of self-disgust.
- **Rescue Remedy** – for calm and general balance.
- **Rock Water** – to address her rigid behavior towards herself.
- **Star of Bethlehem** – to help her traumatized body.
- **Walnut** – to improve her ability to transition from one state to another.
- **Mimulus** – to address her fear of getting fat.
- **Water Violet** – to alleviate her sense of loneliness and disconnection from the world around her.

Sarah scrupulously took the appropriate Bach Flower Remedy dosage and, after a period during which this was combined with other treatments, her situation improved. Today, she is physically and mentally balanced and her weight is completely normal.

11.
ELM

Ulmus procera

FOR TEMPORARY FATIGUE RESULTING FROM THE BURDEN
OF OBLIGATION

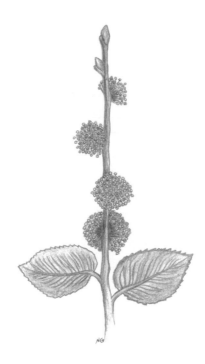

Elm helps diligent, independent children and adolescents who take on a lot of responsibility, do a good job and are proud of their achievements and goals, but burden and exhaust themselves with too many obligations and tasks. A child or adolescent in need of Elm Remedy is naturally generous and will always do what they can to help. Occasionally they take too much on themselves and, when experiencing a sense of temporary weakness which makes them think that the task is difficult and they might fail, will take Elm Remedy to help them calm down and renew their strength.

Elm Remedy can help children and adolescents who take on a lot of responsibility at home and/or in society, and those who participate in many extra-curricular activities or competitions. The Remedy is excellent for children during puberty and is particularly suitable for use during examinations or situations of pressure and stress. It is very important to combine Elm with other Bach Flower Remedies in order to adapt it accurately to the child or adolescent's needs.

Taking the Remedy

Taking the Elm Remedy reminds the child or adolescent to avoid 'carrying the whole world on their shoulders', helps them cope with their work load, and gives them the strength to work energetically and deal with all their tasks with renewed confidence in themselves.

A personal experience

Fourteen-year-old May was a girl who was bright, active and energetic, excelled at her studies, had participated in athletics competitions for the past four years, was a counselor in the scout movement, and volunteered at a sanctuary for abandoned dogs. Her parents sent her to me for help because she had begun to suffer from weakness and fatigue, but refused to give up any of her many activities. When we met, May told me about her beliefs and ambitions in life: 'I want to excel at everything, improve the state of the world, realize all my dreams and succeed, but I'm afraid of failing...' We talked about her desire to fulfill all her ideals and her need to help those who suffer and improve the state of the world, and she realized she needed to let herself relax and rest occasionally.

I prepared a bottle of Bach Flower Remedies for May with the following formula:

- **Elm** – for coping with her tasks in a controlled and balanced way.
- **Rescue Remedy** – for calm and general balance.
- **Olive** – for her mental and physical strength.
- **Walnut** – to improve her ability to move from one situation to another.
- **Mimulus** – to alleviate her fear of failure.
- **Aspen** – to address her hidden fears.
- **Red Chestnut** – for calming and balancing her concern for the whole world.

May tasted the Bach Flower Remedies I prepared for her and scrupulously took the required dose every day. There was an immediate improvement in how she felt and, within a few months, she told me her physical and mental state had improved; she now enjoys success in all areas of her life.

12.
GENTIAN

Gentiana amarelle

FOR FAILURE-RELATED DESPAIR

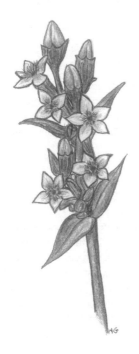

Gentian Remedy is suitable for helping children and adolescents who are in a state of despondency or depression related to temporary failures; it helps them to digest their failures and have the courage to continue to try again. The Remedy helps a child or adolescent who is happy when everything is alright but who tends to be down or depressed when they experience failure. They might lose confidence as a result of failure in class or with their peers, fear exams and refuse to go to school or meet socially with others of their age.

Gentian Remedy helps children and adolescents who easily despair when encountering any difficulty or delay in their studies or in their lives; who view life pessimistically, expect the worst and quickly relinquish their goals after failing and losing self-confidence; and who see their parents' divorce as a failure, feeling torn between their divorced parents. The Remedy is also suitable for helping children and adolescents who tend to get sick and feel despondent at being sick.

Taking the Remedy

Taking Gentian Remedy encourages the child or adolescent, helping them to understand that failure is only a temporary state and life is not a competition. The Remedy encourages faith in oneself and one's personal ability, and reinforces the ability to try again after a failure, to persist and achieve one's goal.

A personal experience

Seventeen-year-old Adam was very successfully learning to drive and enjoyed his lessons. However, he failed his first test. He returned home very dejected and informed his parents that he was giving up on his driving license because he didn't want to do the test again.

His driving teacher called his parents and told them that Adam was an excellent driver and it would be a pity to give up on a driving license because of one failure. I talked to Adam, and prepared a bottle of Bach Flower Remedies for him with the following formula:

🌼 **Gentian** – to cope with the failure he'd experienced, and to reinforce his ability to try again.
🌼 **Rescue Remedy** – for calm and general balance.

- **Walnut** – to improve his ability to transition easily from one state to another.
- **Mimulus** – to reduce his fear of failure.
- **Aspen** – to alleviate his hidden fears.
- **Larch** – to reinforce his self-confidence.
- **White Chestnut** – to soothe the negative thoughts in his mind.

After using the Bach Flower Remedies for several days, Adam agreed to try and drive again, took a few extra lessons and passed the second test very well. He continues to use the formula I gave him, saying that it helps him to calm down and cope with life in the most effective way.

13.
GORSE

Ulex europaeus

FOR DEEP DESPAIR AND HOPELESSNESS

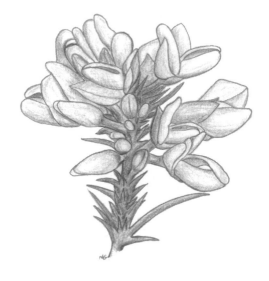

Gorse Remedy helps children and adolescents in states of depression, chronic despair and hopelessness. It is suitable for children and adolescents who have suffered for a long time, and those who have lost the strength to fight and progress in their lives as a result of fear, a painful event, or lengthy illness, and who tend to believe that nothing can be done for them.

Children and adolescents in need of Gorse Remedy have become depressed as a result of many failures or a lengthy illness, and view life with despair, negativity and hopelessness. They believe that they are destined to suffer and tend to say things like: 'There's nothing to be done. I've tried everything; nothing helps...' Despite this, they will allow those who love them to persuade them to try again, even though deep inside, they don't believe they can succeed.

Gorse Remedy can help to improve their mood, encourage them to succeed in their attempts and help them to try any possible way in order to shift their situation and enable them to believe in a better future.

Taking the Remedy

Taking Gorse Remedy can help children and adolescents cope with complicated situations with hope and renewed faith in themselves and the world around them, helping them to find balance, greater strength and a new direction in life, and to open the door to new opportunities.

A personal experience

Ten-year-old Michael arrived in my country with his parents and grandmother and had difficulty making new friends, learning the language and connecting with his new environment. His beloved grandmother died a few months after they arrived and he sank into a depression, fell ill with various illnesses, and didn't want to do anything.

I prepared a bottle of Bach Flower Remedies for Michael with the following formula:

- **Gorse** – for alleviating his chronic depression.
- **Rescue Remedy** – for calm and general balance.
- **Walnut** – for improving his ability to adapt to a variety of situations.

- **Honeysuckle** – to soothe his longing for his grandmother and birth country.
- **Olive** – to strengthen him, body and mind, after his many illnesses.
- **Larch** – to reinforce his self-confidence.
- **Mimulus** – to address his various fears.

When Michael tasted the Remedies, he said happily that the formula tasted like his favorite food, mashed potatoes and peas. After he had used the formula consistently for a few weeks, his condition materially improved and his parents told me that he was beginning to smile, to connect with his peers and even enjoy his lessons at school, and his physical state had improved enormously.

14.
HEATHER

Calluna vulgaris

FOR BEING OVERLY GARRULOUS AND THE DISLIKE OF BEING
ALONE

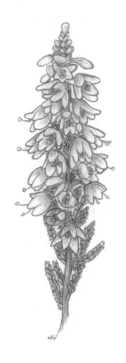

Heather Remedy is suitable for children in great need of attention, who cling physically to a parent or care-giver, dislike being alone, and talk incessantly, telling exaggerated stories about themselves and their parents. Very young children tend to behave in this way as part of a natural and normal transition in childhood, and there is no need to consider this to be a problem as long as this behavior doesn't harm the child or their relations with those around them.

Heather Remedy can help children and adolescents who talk incessantly about themselves, their actions and problems to everyone they meet, even complete strangers, each conversation being about them and their life. They are likely to exhaust anyone around who is listening to them and, since they are unable to listen to anyone else, any conversation with them becomes a never-ending monologue.

A child or adolescent might need Heather Remedy temporarily if they go through a crisis such as an illness, their parents' divorce, a traumatic move from one place to another, a painful parting from a beloved friend or some other trauma.

Taking the Remedy

Taking Heather Remedy helps a child or adolescent to let go of dependency on the company of others, to calm down and moderate the flow of their speech and to be able to listen to others, taking an interest in what they are saying and creating a real and mutual relationship with them.

A personal experience

Twelve-year-old Tammy, whose parents went through a long and painful divorce, was afraid to return home after school and be alone. Every day, she'd go to another friend's home and stay there until late in the evening. At every social meeting, Tammy would talk incessantly about herself and recount intimate details about her parents' divorce. Her mother brought her to me for help, and, although Tammy didn't know me, she started telling me about herself and her life from the moment she entered the room. I prepared a bottle of Bach Flower Remedies for her with the following formula:

- **Heather** – to calm her dependency on the company of others and balance her incessant talking.
- **Rescue Remedy** – for calm and general balance.
- **Star of Bethlehem** – to address the trauma caused by her parents' divorce.
- **Walnut** – to improve her ability to transition easily from one situation to another.
- **Mimulus** – to alleviate her various fears.
- **Aspen** – to alleviate her fear of the unknown future.
- **Larch** – to strengthen her self-confidence.

The moment Tammy took four drops of the Remedies, her incessant talking calmed down. She continued to take the formula and today she is far calmer, is not afraid of being alone at home, her talking has become calmer and more balanced, and she is attentive to what others say.

15.
HOLLY

Ilex aquifolium

FOR SUSPICION, JEALOUSY AND HATRED

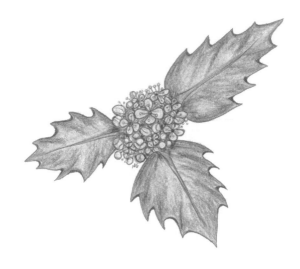

Holly Remedy is suitable for children and adolescents who are filled with feelings of hatred, jealousy, suspicion or revenge and might be dragged into verbal or even physical violence. Young people in need of Holly Remedy tend to be angry and bitter, find fault with others, hold grudges for a long time and share their negative opinions with others. Their inner suffering is considerable and, although in many cases there is no real reason for their misery, they feel stuck, blame others for their suffering, and don't admit that they are angry or jealous. They tend to be suspicious and angry and their hurt feelings may burst out suddenly and aggressively.

Holly Remedy can help address any kind of jealousy throughout childhood, including sibling rivalry and jealousy between friends.

Taking the Remedy

Taking Holly Remedy can help a child or adolescent realize that their negative feelings harm them. The Remedy enables them to stop making themselves miserable and helps them part from feelings of anger and hatred locked up inside them.

A personal experience

Eight-year-old Joseph and nine-year-old Moses were brothers who were jealous of each other and constantly fighting and squabbling. Their exhausted parents told me they had to intervene in their quarrels because they hit each other with great violence and the angry atmosphere at home exhausted the entire family. I talked to each brother individually and prepared a personal bottle of Bach Flower Remedies for each one. Each brother received a formula containing Holly Remedy as well as supplementary Remedies adapted to each one's needs.

The moment each brother took his personal formula, their relationship improved. The two brothers continued to use the Bach Flower Remedies for a long time and their parents told me that by the end of the process, Joseph and Moses had become good friends.

16.
HONEYSUCKLE
Lonicera caprifolium

FOR LONGING AND THINKING ABOUT THE PAST

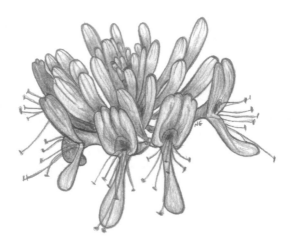

Honeysuckle Remedy is suitable for children and adolescents who are dealing with thoughts about the past, and missing someone or something in their past – for instance, a child who moves from kindergarten to school and is sad, missing both his kindergarten teacher and the kindergarten itself. Honeysuckle Remedy can help with difficulties around parting and difficult transitions for a child or adolescent who suffers from moving from one country to another, moving house or parting from someone beloved who has died.

Children and adolescents can be helped by Honeysuckle Remedy when away from their home and family whom they miss when staying with friends or relatives, or when they are on a trip or at summer camp.

Honeysuckle Remedy helps children and adolescents who are introverted, tend to depression and irritability and who suffer from nightmares resulting from a recurring memory.

Taking the Remedy

Taking Honeysuckle Remedy helps a child or adolescent leave the past behind, live fully in the present, understand lessons they have learned from past experience, and fill them with vitality and energy, enjoying life in the present.

A personal experience

Five-year-old Tom very much wanted to sleep over at his friend Ron's house and the two friends were very happy to go to sleep together. Since this was the first time Tom had slept away from home, he missed his mother and had difficulty falling asleep. Ron's mother called Tom's mother, told her about his difficulties and received permission to help him with a Bach Flower Remedy. Ron's mother put two drops of Honeysuckle and two drops of Rescue Remedy in a glass of water and gave it to Tom to sip. Tom happily drank the water with the Flower Remedies and a few minutes later he calmed down and fell asleep, sleeping deeply and peacefully through the night.

17.
HORNBEAM
Carpinus betulus

FOR DIFFICULTY WAKING UP IN THE MORNING, FATIGUE AND
PROCRASTINATION

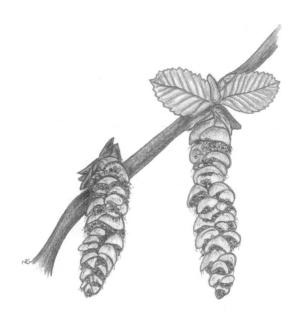

Hornbeam Remedy is suitable for children and adolescents who have difficulty waking and getting up in the morning, feel they have neither the strength nor the desire to deal with daily tasks and life's routine, and who are tired at the very thought of the tasks they have to carry out. They feel tired and bored, and put off doing their tasks for as long as possible, preferring to sink into sleep.

These sensations of fatigue and dejection usually stem from boredom or a fundamental dissatisfaction with their life, which leads to chronic procrastination. When they are helped to start taking action, their fatigue disappears, they are full of energy and happiness, and they tend to carry out their tasks with joy and satisfaction.

Hornbeam Remedy can help children and adolescents who suffer from sensations of vagueness and heaviness, who have difficulty getting up in the morning and going to school, and who feel emotionally tired after excitement, tension, a holiday or illness, and have difficulty going back to kindergarten or school.

Taking the Remedy

Taking Hornbeam Remedy can help a child or adolescent to relieve fatigue; rouse renewed interest in life, giving them the strength to complete their daily tasks; and foster their ability to cope with difficulties and complete their assignments.

A personal experience

One of the first people to come to me for help was 13-year-old Roy, whose mother approached me. Roy had great difficulty getting up in the morning, and he felt tired and lacking in energy during the day. He tended to put off doing homework, assignments for school, tidying his room, etc. His mother had to wake him every morning and remind him repeatedly of what he had to do. When I asked him how he felt, he looked down, saying, 'I'm just tired all the time. I'm bored, and I don't feel like doing anything...'

I prepared a bottle of Bach Flower Remedies for Roy with the following formula:

- ❀ **Hornbeam** – to improve his procrastination and inability to wake up in the morning.
- ❀ **Rescue Remedy** – for calm and general balance.
- ❀ **Walnut** – to improve his ability to transition easily from a state of sleep to one of wakefulness.
- ❀ **Olive** – for his mental and physical reinforcement.
- ❀ **Wild Oat** – to find and manifest his calling.
- ❀ **Larch** – for strengthening his faith in himself and his abilities.
- ❀ **Mimulus** – to alleviate his fear of failing to carry out assignments.

After taking the Remedies for several days, Roy managed to wake up in the morning by himself and, about two months later, I met him and his mother in my clinic. Roy's mother told me that his behavior at school was wonderfully improved and Roy looked at me, saying, 'I wanted to say thank you very much. I used to be tired and depressed all the time, and now I have strength and energy, and I enjoy doing all sorts of things.' I was very moved and thanked him for his warm words.

Roy was one of the first children who showed me that, with the help of Bach Flower Remedies, their life could change for the better in a most significant way. He continued to use Bach Flower Remedies for many years, every time he felt he needed help.

18.
IMPATIENS
Impatiens glandulifera

FOR IMPATIENCE

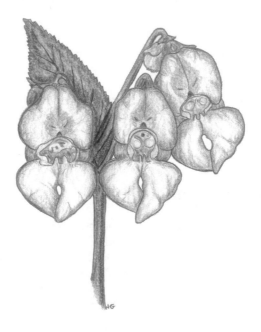

Impatiens Remedy is suitable for children and adolescents who are agile, alert, quick thinking and active, who know what they want and are keen for things to be done fast. They tend to be impatient, always on the move and, when things don't progress at the pace they wish, tend to blame others. They are driven by restlessness and are capable of seeing things in a flash and making serious decisions before someone else can take a breath. They are self-reliant and often tend to take too much on themselves and, when exhausted, become angry and irritable.

Children and adolescents in need of Impatiens Remedy are full of anger when things don't happen the way they want them to, saying 'Move over, let me do it'. They prefer to work alone at their own quick pace, find fault with others and tend to outbursts of anger and quarrels when things don't work out as they wish.

Impatiens Remedy also helps children and adolescents who suffer from tension, irritability, muscle spasms in the back and neck, nocturnal tooth-grinding, upset stomach, skin disorders and physical and mental pain.

Taking the Remedy

Taking Impatiens Remedy helps children and adolescent to relax, develop empathy and tolerance for the flaws in others, and accept an existing situation and work according to a natural life rhythm that suits their body and mind.

A personal experience

Six-year-old Lily sat in front of me, nervously biting her nails. Her parents brought her to me because she suffered from irritability and bad stomach pains. She had undergone comprehensive medical tests that found no physical reason for the pain. Lily had difficulty sitting quietly at home and in the classroom, and when I asked her when it was that she suffered from stomach pain, she said that when she was tired and irritable her belly began to hurt.

I prepared a bottle of Bach Flower Remedies for Lily with the following formula:

- **Impatiens** – to address her tension, irritability and restlessness.
- **Rescue Remedy** – for calm and general balance.
- **Crab Apple** – for mental and physical cleansing and to calm her stomachaches.
- **Walnut** – to strengthen her ability to transition easily from one situation to another.
- **Mimulus** – for her fear of the pain bombarding her.
- **Aspen** – for her fear of the unknown.

When Lily tasted the formula I had prepared for her, she smiled, saying, 'It tastes like an almond croissant!' A week later, her mother told me that she was calmer, and had significantly fewer stomach pains.

After Lily had taken the Bach Flower Remedies consistently for about three months, we met again in my clinic. She sat calm and smiling in front of me, and her parents told me that her stomach pains had vanished, she was calmer and was capable of sitting in class for a long time.

Lily continues to take the Bach Flower Remedies whenever she feels the need, and still thinks they taste like almond croissants…

19.
LARCH

Larix decidua

FOR INSECURITY AND LACK OF SELF-ESTEEM

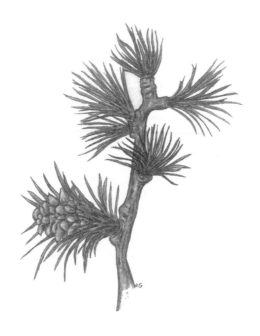

Larch Remedy is suitable for children and adolescents who suffer from a lack of self-confidence and are afraid they won't be able to do things like others around them. They are afraid of failing, and sometimes their lack of confidence may paralyze them and prevent them from even trying to do something, so they need a great deal of encouragement and reinforcement from their parents, teachers and friends.

Larch Remedy can help a hesitant child or adolescent who feels they can't do things well by him/herself and who often say, 'I can't...' These young people tend to have a low self-image and when they succeed in something, they will allow someone else to pick the fruits of their success because they'd often rather take a back seat and let others bask in the limelight, even when they are actually less successful.

Larch Remedy is also suitable for helping children and adolescents who are strong, successful and talented but who have temporarily lost their self-confidence because of life circumstances.

Taking the Remedy

Taking Larch Remedy builds and reinforces self-confidence, helping children and adolescents to learn to appreciate themselves, to cope with difficult and stressful situations, to do things they are afraid of, and to acknowledge their strengths and abilities.

A personal experience

Thirteen-year-old Mika's teacher set up a meeting with Mika and her parents. She told them about a new school project intended to encourage creative children, and suggested that Mika join a special group, where the children would receive supervision and special lessons on the subject of art. Mika was afraid that her drawings weren't good enough, and said 'I very much want to join the group, but the other children are much better than I am... I just can't do it.' Mika's parents asked me to help strengthen Mika's self-esteem and, after talking to her, I prepared a bottle of Bach Flower Remedies with the following formula:

- **Larch** – for strengthening her self-confidence.
- **Walnut** – for improving her ability to successfully join a new group.
- **Mimulus** – for alleviating her fear of failure.

- **Aspen** – for relieving her fear of the unknown.
- **Rescue Remedy** – for calm and general balance.
- **Wild Oat** – to help her find her creative path.
- **White Chestnut** – to calm her negative thoughts about herself.

After taking the Remedies for a week, Mika decided to join the art group and today she greatly enjoys creativity and painting with her friends.

20.
MIMULUS

Mimulus guttatus

FOR FEARS AND ANXIETY

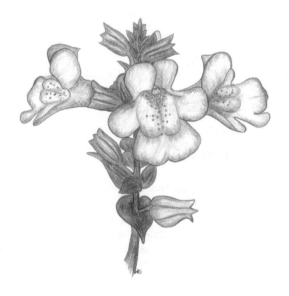

Mimulus Remedy is suitable for children and adolescents who suffer from fear of something known, such as exams, visiting the dentist, elevators, flying, certain animals, etc – a fear that overwhelms them and restricts their activities. Children and adolescents in need of Mimulus Remedy tend to be naturally nervous, unconfident, very sensitive to noise and, occasionally, tend to quarrel easily.

As a result of humanity's massive transition to an urban environment, many children and adolescents tend to fear a lot of animals, being out in nature, and natural phenomena such as lightning and thunder. In addition, many children and adolescents are exposed to frightening films, as a result of which they develop fears that, in previous years, weren't common among young people. Covid-19 has added new fears to our lives. Many children and adolescents have started being afraid of illness and medical problems and Mimulus Remedy can help reduce their various fears. It also helps children and adolescents who suffer from shortness of breath, sinus problems, sensations of tightness in the throat, chills and tremors in the body.

Taking the Remedy

Mimulus Remedy can help children and adolescents release their fears; it gives them the strength and courage to cope with difficult issues, and enables them to live their life fully and act without fear.

A personal experience

Eight-year-old Natalie really liked candies and, as a result, suffered from a lot of holes in her teeth. Her mother took her to a dentist who specialized in treating children, but Natalie was very frightened of him. Every time she visited the dentist for treatment, her whole body trembled, she cried, screamed and refused to sit in the dentist's chair. Her mother asked for my help and, after talking to them both, I prepared a bottle of Bach Flower Remedies for Natalie with the following formula:

- **Mimulus** – to reduce her fear of the dentist.
- **Rescue Remedy** – for calm and general balance.
- **Aspen** – to calm her hidden fears.
- **Walnut** – to improve her ability to transition from one situation to another.

This formula was meant to be taken only the week before and during Natalie's dental treatments. Her mother told me that, due to the Bach Flower Remedies, Natalie was very calm before the treatment and agreed to climb into the dentist's chair and sit there quietly. She asked to hold the bottle of Bach Flower Remedies during the treatment, and every time she felt her fear growing, the doctor allowed her to take a few drops from the bottle.

The dental appointment went successfully and everyone wondered at Natalie's mature, calm behavior. At the end of the treatment, she said to the dentist: 'I'm brave and I'm not afraid of you anymore. We're friends.'

Natalie and her mother continue to use the bottle of Bach Flower Remedies when needed, and both enjoy the results.

21.
MUSTARD
Sinapis arvensis

FOR SUDDEN DEPRESSION AND DESPAIR

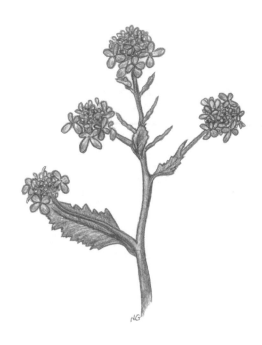

Mustard Remedy is suitable for children and adolescents who suffer from depression that appears suddenly without any obvious reason, causing a great deal of suffering.

This deep depression passes and disappears just as it arrived and, to the child or adolescent, these attacks seem to come out of nowhere. The depression appears in waves that are impossible to predict and the young person has no control over them.

When a child or adolescent finds they have these signs of depression, *they should be referred to a conventional doctor for treatment immediately*, and use Mustard Remedy as a supplement, in coordination with the conventional doctor treating them.

Mustard Remedy can also help a child or adolescent who is suffering from hormonal problems and depression that stems from a hormonal imbalance, and problems with balance, dizziness and sudden mood swings.

Taking the Remedy

Taking Mustard Remedy can bring relief to the child or adolescent, improving their mood and mental and physical balance, enabling them to find a way to emerge from the depression.

A personal experience

Fifteen-year-old Daniela suffered greatly from bouts of depression that appeared in waves, causing her to retreat, avoiding the company of even the people closest to her. The psychologist who treated her recommended she come and see me and we met in the clinic for a conversation. Daniela told me that the depression appeared without any reason, saying: 'I suffer from depression and am disgusted by myself because I have a lot of acne and heavy bleeding when I menstruate, and I don't want to be near other people and disgust them too.'

I prepared a bottle of Bach Flower Remedies for Daniela with the following formula:

- **Mustard** – for addressing her depression and hormonal imbalance.
- **Rescue Remedy** – for calm and general balance.
- **Walnut** – to improve her ability to emerge from the depression.
- **Crab Apple** – to address her self-disgust at her acne and menstruation problems.
- **Larch** – to strengthan her self-confidence.
- **Water Violet** – for addressing her tendency to avoid people.
- **Mimulus** – to calm her various fears.

In order to help Daniela with her acne, I prepared a treatment spray for her with the following formula:

- **Rescue Remedy** – to calm her skin and for general balance.
- **Crab Apple** – to clean her skin and address her sense of self-disgust.
- **Cherry Plum** – to counteract the flare-ups of acne that sometimes appeared overnight.
- **Walnut** – to improve her ability to transition in the best way possible from one situation to another.
- **Mustard** – to address the hormonal cause of the appearance of acne.

I advised Daniela to use the bottle of Bach Flower Remedies and the treatment spray every day, and after a short time there was a noticeable improvement in her condition. After persevering for several months with the help of the Bach Flower Remedy formula at the same time as the conventional treatment with her psychologist, Daniela told me her depression had mostly passed, her menstruation was balanced, her skin had significantly improved and she enjoyed spending time with her family and friends.

22.
OAK

Quercus robur

FOR ENDURANCE AND SUPPORTING CHALLENGING EFFORT

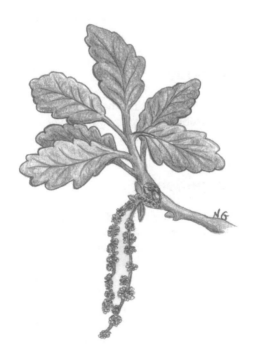

Oak Remedy is suitable for supporting children and adolescents with a strong personality, who work hard and physically and mentally exhaust themselves. They are courageous, strong fighters who have difficulty being flexible, and are steadfast in their fight and struggle during an event or illness, refusing to surrender even when all hope is lost.

They strive and battle with difficulties and, when life seems to be a long, exhausting struggle, they fight against all odds, tending to blame themselves when there is no improvement in their situation. They hide their tiredness from others, complain very rarely, and might exhaust themselves even when it's unnecessary and ineffective. They may suffer from constipation, tiredness and chronic illness.

Children and adolescents in need of Oak Remedy view their studies as an obligation that must be carried out at any price in the best possible way, sometimes because their ambitious parents push them to study and succeed in any situation. They have apparently inexhaustible reserves of strength and only rarely will they ask for help or advice.

Taking the Remedy

Taking Oak Remedy encourages the child or adolescent to develop mental and practical flexibility, recognize when they should stop driving themselves, and learn there is no need to fight all the time.

A personal experience

Nine-year-old Nathan excelled at his studies and after achievement tests held at his school, it was suggested to his parents that he move to a higher class, where he'd study with children who were two years older than him. He studied hard in the new class, but after two months he began to suffer from a chronic runny nose and a troublesome cough and his parents brought him to me for help. After talking for some time, Nathan admitted that he was making an effort to study because he felt he had to excel and succeed, but it was hard for him being the smallest boy in class, and he missed his friends from his previous class and was unable to connect with students in the new class.

I prepared a bottle of Bach Flower Remedies for Nathan with the following formula:

- **Oak** – to encourage and develop mental and practical flexibility in his studies.
- **Rescue Remedy** – for calm and general balance.
- **Walnut** – to improve his ability to adjust to his new situation.
- **Olive** – for physical and mental reinforcement.
- **Water Violet** – to address his sense of loneliness in the new class.
- **Honeysuckle** – to address his longing for his friends in his previous class.
- **Mimulus** – to address his fears of failure and loneliness.

Nathan's parents gave him the formula four times a day, occasionally adding it to his water bottle. After about three weeks, his chronic runny nose ceased and he felt positive and full of energy. After about three months, his parents told me that he had connected with children in his new class and was very happy in their company.

23.
OLIVE

Olea europaca

FOR EXTREME FATIGUE AND MENTAL EXHAUSTION

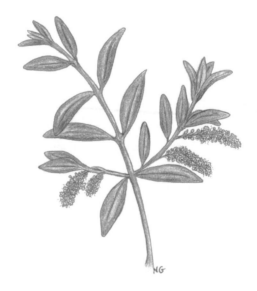

Olive Remedy is suitable for reinforcing mental and physical strength in children and adolescents during an illness or for recovery from a difficult illness. It is also a suitable supplement for children and adolescents in situations of extreme body-mind exhaustion; after a great and sustained effort as a result of hard mental and physical work; after a lengthy illness; or when they are suffering from chronic illness. Olive Remedy is a suitable supplement during challenging physical treatments such as chemotherapy, and during difficult, exhausting, emotional transitions.

A child or adolescent in need of Olive Remedy feels exhausted and doesn't have the strength to go on; they might suffer from various allergies, and to them, life appears difficult, exhausting and without pleasure.

Many children and adolescents suffer from physical exhaustion after having Covid-19 and Olive Remedy can help them to recover in the best possible way.

Taking the Remedy

Taking Olive Remedy is refreshing and strengthening. It restores the child or adolescent, strengthening body and mind, helping them to recover, renew their strength and be refilled with vitality and energy.

A personal experience

Eleven-year-old Emanuel, who was recovering from Covid-19, felt physically and mentally exhausted. He suffered from loss of hair, skin problems and various fears. I prepared a bottle of Bach Flower Remedies for him with the following formula:

- **Olive** – for mental and physical strength and to rehabilitate his body after the illness.
- **Rescue Remedy** – for calm and general balance.
- **Star of Bethlehem** – to alleviate his physical and mental trauma caused by the illness.
- **Walnut** – for protection and to improve his ability to transition easily from one situation to another.
- **Mimulus** – to alleviate his conscious fears.
- **Aspen** – to address his hidden fears.

🌸 **Crab Apple** – to address his skin problems and to facilitate his physical and mental cleansing.

After using the bottle of Bach Flower Remedies consistently for about three weeks, there was a significant improvement in Emanuel's physical and mental condition and he continued to use Bach Flower Remedies until he had completely recovered.

24.
PINE

Pinus sylvestris

FOR A TENDENCY TO SELF-BLAME

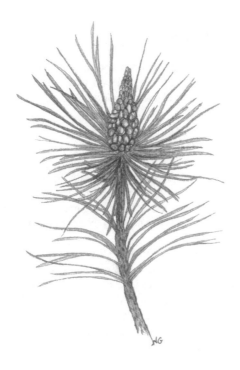

Pine Remedy is suitable for idealistic children and adolescents who set themselves a very high standard of behavior and performance and who suffer from self-blame, heartache and depression when they fail to meet their own requirements. They overburden themselves out of a sense of obligation and personal responsibility and, when a project in which they are involved fails, they tend to get angry, mainly blaming themselves, even if it fails as a result of the mistakes of others. When their group is blamed, they take responsibility for the faults of others and accept the punishment without complaint.

Children and adolescents in need of Pine Remedy blame themselves for mistakes they made in the past and are severe with themselves regarding any little error they make, which evokes a sense of despair. They tend to relinquish their share of praise or reward, constantly apologizing and feeling tired and depressed.

Taking the Remedy

Taking Pine Remedy allows children and adolescents to relate to the issue of responsibility in a more balanced way, encouraging their ability to forgive themselves and observe their actions objectively and calmly.

A personal experience

Five-year-old Sharon came home very sad from kindergarten, didn't want to eat her lunch, and shut herself in her room. When her mother asked her what had happened, she burst into tears and told her that Dana, her best friend, had hurt herself in the kindergarten and been taken to the clinic.

'It all happened because of me... We were playing near the swing, Dana ran after me and I managed to run away, but she got hit hard by the swing... and she was bleeding... and it was all my fault...' Sharon's mother explained to her that it wasn't her fault, things like that can happen, but Sharon continued feeling very sad. Her mother called me, told me that Sharon was very upset and asked me to prepare a bottle of Bach Flower Remedies for her. Which I did with the following formula:

🌼 **Pine** – to alleviate her feelings of guilt.
🌼 **Rescue Remedy** – for calm and general balance.

🌸 **Walnut** – to improve her ability to move easily from one situation to another.

🌸 **Mimulus** – to address her fears at what had happened to her friend.

🌸 **Aspen** – to alleviate her hidden fears related to the situation.

The bottle of Bach Flower Remedies was meant to help with the specific situation and Sharon calmed down immediately after tasting the Remedy. Her mother continued to give it to her for about a week, until she saw that Sharon had completely calmed down.

25.
RED CHESTNUT
Aesculus carnea

FOR OVERLY DEEP CONCERN FOR THE
WELFARE OF OTHERS

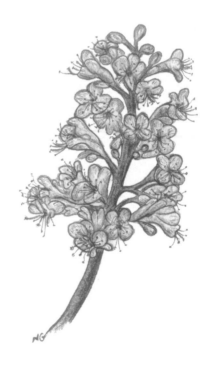

Red Chestnut Remedy is suitable for children and adolescents who are very anxious about the health and wellbeing of others. They are tense, anxious and emotionally burdened, frequently afraid that those they love will have an accident or fall ill.

They always imagine the worst, are very troubled by reports of illness or tragedy and their actions may reflect their parents' or caretakers' behavioral patterns. They tend to identify with the suffering of others, and feel helpless when they cannot help or relieve the suffering of people or animals in faraway places.

Adding Red Chestnut Remedy to the personal formula of attentive, conscientious children and adolescents who are aware of the state of the earth and concerned because of the climate crisis and ecological and social problems in our world, can calm their fears, enabling them to act according to their conscience in a calmer, more balanced way.

Red Chestnut Remedy can help a child who has been given great responsibility at a young age, such as caring for a younger sibling, helping a disabled parent or caring for many animals.

Taking the Remedy

Taking Red Chestnut Remedy can help children and adolescents to calm down, release the 'horror movies' in their head, and take care of those they love in a way that is balanced and calm, without hysteria, pressure, fear or anxiety.

A personal experience

Nine-year-old Ariel was his mother's only child and they had no close family. His mother told me that lately Ariel had tended to call her often during the day to ask her how she was. He clung to her from the moment she returned from work, and at bedtime, he had difficulty parting from her and falling asleep. When the three of us met and talked, Ariel told us that the mother of one of his friends had died, and the father of the friend was taking care of him and his brother.

Ariel said to his mother: 'I worry about you all the time and I'm afraid something bad could happen to you… I don't have a father or a brother to take care of me and if something happens to you, I will be all on my own…' Ariel's mother told him that she'd prepared a legal document with her best friend who had promised to take care of Ariel if the need arose.

I prepared a bottle of Bach Flower Remedies for Ariel with the following formula:

- **Red Chestnut** – for calming his concern and fear for his mother's wellbeing.
- **Rescue Remedy** – for calm and general balance.
- **Mimulus** – to alleviate his fear of being alone in the world, without his mother.
- **Aspen** – to alleviate his hidden fears.
- **Larch** – to reinforce his self-confidence.
- **Walnut** – to improve his ability to move from one situation to another.
- **White Chestnut** – to calm his troubling thoughts.

Once Ariel began to take the Bach Flower formula, his fears relaxed, and every time he started to worry, he would run to the fridge to take 6 drops from the Remedy bottle I had prepared for him.

26.
ROCK ROSE

Helianthemum nummularium

FOR PANIC, TERROR AND ANXIETY ATTACKS

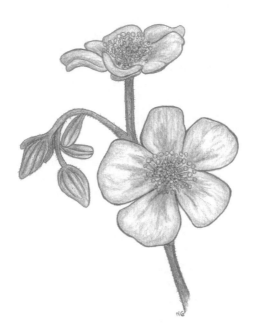

Rock Rose Remedy can help children and adolescents in states of extreme fear, hysteria, 'black out', terror or panic, or a paralyzing attack of anxiety. It is intended to treat acute conditions of fear and extreme anxiety, *and should not be used as a treatment remedy for long periods of time*.

Rock Rose Remedy is commonly used in combination with other suitable Remedies in order to create a one-off formula for children or adolescents who are suffering from exam anxiety, paralyzing anxiety attacks, hysteria or nightmares from which they wake up screaming.

Rock Rose Remedy is a component in Rescue Remedy, Dr Edward Bach's formula for treating emergency situations, and is suitable for immediate use after a traumatic, frightening and shocking event.

Taking the Remedy

Taking the Rock Rose Remedy can help children and adolescents calm down and find balance, encourage them, soothe their anxieties and give them the courage required to overcome their fears and act calmly when in distress.

A personal experience

One-year-old Ethan's mother told me that he occasionally woke up in the middle of the night sobbing and completely drenched in sweat. Although she would run to him and hug him, it would take time for him to stop screaming and crying.

I prepared a bottle of Bach Flower Remedies for Ethan with the following formula, intended only for those moments when he woke screaming:

- **Rock Rose** – to calm his fears and anxieties.
- **Rescue Remedy** – for calm and general balance.
- **Walnut** – to improve his ability to calm down and for general protection.
- **Aspen** – to address his hidden fears.
- **Mimulus** – to address his concrete fears.

Ethan's mother told me that she'd given him 4 drops from the bottle every time he woke up sobbing in alarm and he'd immediately calmed down. After a while, he stopped waking up during the night, but she keeps the bottle in the fridge in case it is needed.

27.
ROCK WATER

Aqua petra

FOR ALLEVIATING RIGID SELF-DISCIPLINE

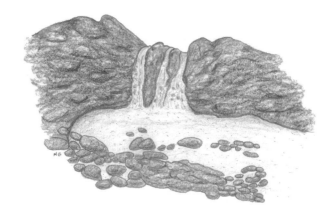

Rock Water is suitable for children and adolescents with rigid self-discipline, who demand perfection of themselves and don't allow anything to distract them from their purpose. They have high ideals that they adhere to and they tend to be strict and demanding of themselves. They maintain a strict diet and/or physical fitness. They are intolerant, full of self-criticism, but will rarely openly criticize others.

Rock Water Remedy can also help with various eating disorders, constipation and behavioral problems in children and adolescents. It is suitable for supporting children and adolescents who are consistently engaged in sports, or compete in their or their parents' favorite sport.

Rock Water is the only Remedy that Dr Bach did not formulate from flowers, but from the waters of Sotwell Spring.

Taking the Remedy

Taking Rock Water Remedy can help a child or adolescent to calm down, soften, and enjoy spontaneity and mental and physical flexibility.

A personal experience

Thirteen-year-old Liam loved sport, participated in his school rowing team, trained several times a week, and made sure he ate properly. He and his parents came to see me after he sprained his ankle and refused to rest, though he did agree to receive help so he could recover quickly and return to his training routine.

I prepared a bottle of Bach Flower Remedies for Liam with the following formula:

- **Rock Water** – to help him calm down, be more flexible and enable himself to rest and recover.
- **Rescue Remedy** – for calm and general balance.
- **Walnut** – to improve his ability to move from one situation to another.
- **Mimulus** – to address his fear of becoming unfit because of the break in his training.
- **Aspen** – to relieve his hidden fears.
- **Oak** – to relieve his tendency to train and exhaust himself despite his injured ankle.

* **Olive** – for reinforcement of body and mind and to encourage the recovery of his sprained ankle.

In addition, I prepared a cream for him to rub into the injured area with the following formula:

* **Rock Water** – to help the area become more relaxed and flexible.
* **Rescue Remedy** – for calm and general balance.
* **Star of Bethlehem** – to relieve the trauma in his injured ankle.
* **Crab Apple** – for deep cleansing and absorption of the cream into his skin.
* **Walnut** – to improve his ability to move easily from one situation to another.

Liam scrupulously took 6 drops of the Bach Flower Remedy four times a day, and rubbed the cream into the injured area as needed. He became calmer, his condition improved quickly, and his ankle recovered amazingly well.

28.
SCLERANTHUS

Scleranthus annus

FOR MOOD SWINGS AND DIFFICULTY MAKING DECISIONS

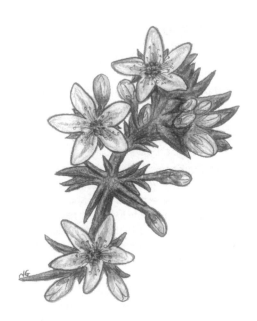

Scleranthus Remedy is suitable for children and adolescents who have difficulty making decisions, are hesitant, procrastinate excessively, and suffer from mood swings and internal arguments. In most cases, these young people tend not to share their dilemmas with others or ask for advice, they might suffer from instability, lack of self-confidence, lack of concentration and restlessness. Their moods are jumpy and even after they make a decision, they could change their mind.

Scleranthus Remedy can help children and adolescents who suffer from travel sickness, neurological problems and/or ear problems. It is suitable for children and adolescents who suffer from the 'wandering pain' syndrome during illness, when the pain keeps appearing in a different part of the body and the symptoms vary in the extreme: constipation followed by diarrhea, high fever followed by very low temperature, hunger followed by complete loss of appetite, etc.

Taking the Remedy

Taking Scleranthus Remedy can help children and adolescents focus and learn to connect emotion and logic, so they can make the best decisions fast, and find physical and mental stability and equilibrium.

A personal experience

Fifteen-year-old Ruth came to me for treatment and told me that she was going through a period of difficult deliberation regarding her continued studies and, although many advised her, she couldn't wholeheartedly accept their advice. She suffered from many fears, a lack of confidence, and lightning mood swings. In addition, she had begun to suffer from dizziness that had no medical explanation, despite many investigations.

I prepared a bottle of Bach Flower Remedies for Ruth with the following formula:

- **Scleranthus** – to improve her physical and mental equilibrium, and her ability to arrive at good decisions for herself.
- **Rescue Remedy** – for calm and general balance.
- **Walnut** – for protection and to improve her ability to move easily from one situation to another.

- **Larch** – to reinforce her self-confidence.
- **Mimulus** – to alleviate her concrete fears.
- **Aspen** – to alleviate her hidden fears.
- **Wild Oat** – to help her find her calling in life.

Ruth loved the Bach Flower Remedies I prepared for her and kept the bottle close to her. Two weeks later, she told me she'd decided which course of study to choose and, after two and a half months, she joyfully told me that, since she'd begun using Bach Flower Remedies, her dizziness had stopped, her fears had calmed down and she was feeling a lot more confident.

29.
STAR OF BETHLEHEM
Ornithogalum umbellatum

FOR PHYSICAL AND MENTAL SHOCK

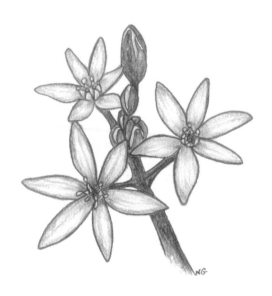

Star of Bethlehem Remedy can help children and adolescents who suffer from grief, numbness, emotional and physical shock and deep-rooted problems stemming from trauma they have experienced. The Remedy also treats old traumas and can help children and adolescents who have suffered from neglect or abuse.

The Remedy is suitable for addressing emergency situations in the life of a child or adolescent, as it neutralizes the shock element in difficult or traumatic events and enables full recovery.

The Star of Bethlehem Remedy is included in Rescue Remedy in order to help in situations of physical and mental shock, trauma and accidents.

Taking the Remedy

Taking the Star of Bethlehem Remedy can help a child or adolescent release physical and mental blocks, restore equilibrium, see problems clearly, find peace and comfort, calm down and heal.

A personal experience

Three-month-year-old Lucy experienced a complicated birth. She cried day and night, had difficulty sleeping and suffered from stomachaches.

Her parents added 6 drops of the following formula to her bath water:

- **Star of Bethlehem** – to address the trauma of her birth.
- **Walnut** – for protection and to improve her ability to move easily from one situation to another.
- **Rescue Remedy** – for calm and general balance.

After a few days, during which she enjoyed a daily bath with the Bach Flower Remedies, Lucy's condition improved significantly and her parents told me that she was calmer and more cheerful.

30.
SWEET CHESTNUT

Castanea sativa

FOR DEEP DESPAIR AND EXTREME MENTAL ANGUISH

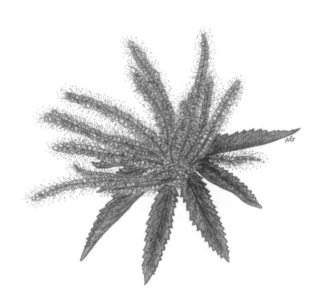

Sweet Chestnut Remedy can help children and adolescents who are very depressed or utterly in despair, who retreat and weep wordlessly, their anxiety and pain so great they feel they cannot bear the existing situation any longer.

Children and adolescents are in need of Sweet Chestnut when they feel their body and mind are betraying them, when their despair increases and the mental torment is so great they cannot bear it, feeling that they've reached their limit. They cannot speak or even pray for help.

Sweet Chestnut can be given to a child or adolescent who is suffering from emotional torment and profound depression as a result of a difficult event like their parents' divorce, severe illness or grief, when they try to hide their distress from others and are silent.

Taking the Remedy

Taking Sweet Chestnut Remedy can help a child or adolescent reinforce their faith in themselves and understand that an end to suffering and torment is in sight, which can restore hope to their life.

A personal experience

When six-year-old Sean's parents told him they were getting a divorce, he burst into tears and tried to persuade them to stay together. For days, Sean begged his parents again and again not to get divorced, promising them that he'd be good and do whatever they asked him to do, as long as they stayed together. His parents explained to him that, although they were all sad, they weren't happy together, and they were definitely getting a divorce.

Sean started to withdraw, turning into a sad and silent child. His parents brought him to me for help and, only after a very long conversation, did he agree to tell me what was troubling him. I prepared a bottle of Bach Flower Remedies for Sean with the following formula:

- **Sweet Chestnut** – to relieve his deep suffering.
- **Rescue Remedy** – for calm and general balance.
- **Walnut** – to improve his ability to move easily from one situation to another.

- **Mimulus** – to address his concrete fears about the divorce and its consequences.
- **Aspen** – to address his hidden fears.
- **Red Chestnut** – to address his fears of something bad happening to those he loved.
- **Larch** – to strengthen his self-confidence.

After taking the Bach Flower Remedies, Sean calmed down and even began to talk about what he was going through. Later on, I adjusted the formula with another that was suitable for his changing condition.

Sean continued to use Bach Flower Remedies for a long time, and said they really helped him.

31.
VERVAIN

Verbena officinalis

FOR EXTREME ENTHUSIASM

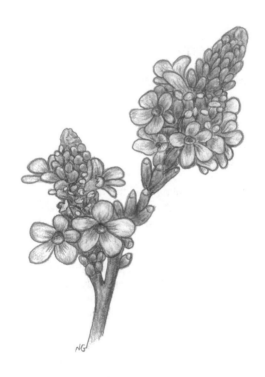

Vervain Remedy is suitable for children and adolescents who are impulsive and idealistic with a strong will, ready to face any challenge and to work hard. They are quick-thinking and agile, refuse to change their opinions, enjoy fighting and arguing, always want to fight for justice, and insist on standing their ground when anyone else would have given up. They tend to be fixed in their beliefs and, since they are motivated by devotion and concern for others and by a passion to inspire others to change, they try with all their power, determinedly and enthusiastically, to persuade those around them to believe in their way.

They are mentally and physically inflexible and tend to interfere in the affairs of others. As a result of their untiring efforts, they are constantly under pressure, suffering from anxiety and stress, and tend to be tense and frustrated and, occasionally, hyperactive. They need less sleep than other children and sometimes suffer from difficulty sleeping.

Taking the Remedy

Taking Vervain Remedy can help children and adolescents to calm and balance their will power, and to be able to listen to others and respect their opinions.

A personal experience

Twelve-year-old Leah saw a film about the hardships of animals and decided to become vegan. Greatly enjoying vegan food, she was determined to persuade everyone she knew to become vegan. At every possible opportunity, she would lecture her family and friends on the state of the world, the suffering of animals and the huge importance of veganism. She spent every free moment on this issue, attending demonstrations and lectures, becoming physically and mentally stressed and exhausted yet unable to fall asleep.

I prepared a bottle of Bach Flower Remedies for Leah with the following formula:

- **Vervain** – to balance her will power and moderate her 'lectures'.
- **Rescue Remedy** – for calm and general balance.
- **Walnut** – to improve her ability to move easily from one subject to another.

- **Red Chestnut** – to moderate her extreme concern for animals and the world.
- **Aspen** – to address her hidden fears.
- **Mimulus** – to address her concrete fears.
- **White Chestnut** – to calm her endless thoughts and improve her ability to fall asleep.

After taking Bach Flower Remedies for three weeks, Leah told me that she was feeling calmer, her emotional state had improved and she was managing to sleep. She continues to be vegan and to work for the world and for animals, but she no longer exhausts those around her or herself.

32.
VINE
Vitis vinifera

FOR ALLEVIATING THE DESIRE TO CONTROL
EVERY SITUATION

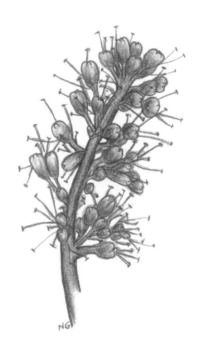

Vine Remedy can help children and adolescents who are natural leaders, who are sure of themselves and believe they know better than everyone else so that, in their opinion, everyone needs to listen to them and do as they say. They tend to have an excessively strong will and ambition, to be stubborn and intolerant, and occasionally aggressive. They are authoritative, always striving to lead others and, since they tend to be aggressive, they have the potential to become a bully. Children and adolescents in need of Vine Remedy might be cruel, controlling and domineering, undermine others and assume authority at their expense. They don't argue but give their opinion, expecting it to be accepted without question. At the same time, they show initiative in every situation, and in an emergency, will lead others out of difficult situations.

Taking the Remedy

Taking Vine Remedy can help a child or adolescent balance their will power, enabling them to learn to respect others, to combine authority, compassion and understanding, to be more flexible and to allow others to express themselves and grow in their own way.

A personal experience

Four-year-old Rebecca insisted on having her own way; she would only eat certain foods; she was afraid of the dark and insisted they leave lights on in the house. Every evening, she informed her parents that she was staying up to watch her favorite TV programs and refused to shower and go to sleep at the appointed time. Every morning, she dilly-dallied over choosing her clothes by herself. She was the leader at kindergarten, and when her friend, May, didn't obey her, she hit her, telling the other children in the kindergarten: 'You're not allowed to play with May. She's disgusting'. Rebecca's parents brought her to me for help and, after talking to them and to Rebecca, I prepared a bottle of Bach Flower Remedies for her with the following formula:

- 🌸 **Vine** – to address her tendency to try to control everyone.
- 🌸 **Rescue Remedy** – for calm and general balance.
- 🌸 **Walnut** – to improve her ability to move easily from one situation to another.

🌺 **Rock Water** – to address her rigidity and stubbornness.
🌺 **Crab Apple** – to address her avoidance of many foods.
🌺 **Mimulus** – to address her fear of the dark.
🌺 **Aspen** – to address her hidden fears.

Rebecca loved the Bach Flower Remedies she was given and after a week her mother joyfully called me to say that Rebecca had changed for the better.

After taking the Remedies for about two and a half months, her parents told me that Rebecca's behavior at home and at kindergarten was exemplary, her fears had passed and she had learned to consider others.

33.
WALNUT

Juglans regia

FOR PROTECTION AND ADDRESSING DIFFICULTY ADJUSTING

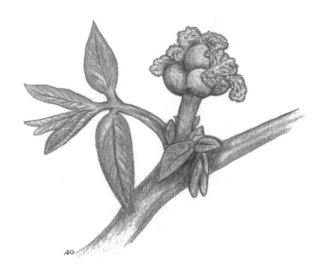

Walnut Remedy can help children of all ages to cope successfully with life transitions from the moment of birth and their entry into the world, helping them to pass calmly and confidently from one stage to another. Walnut Remedy is suitable for helping children and adolescents who have difficulty adjusting to new situations, such as: moving to a new kindergarten/school, home or country; physical changes, such as: teething in babies, weaning, the start of adolescence, menstruation, etc.

Walnut Remedy can help children and adolescents in situations of sorrow and pain after events like their parents' divorce or the death of someone close, because it helps them to overcome difficulties at this stage of their life and move on. It can also help them to dare to change significant things in their life, break behavioral patterns that no longer serve them, relinquish bad habits or substances to which they are addicted, re-invent their life and fulfill their dreams in the best possible way.

In today's world, many children and adolescents spend most of their time looking at the screens of mobile phones, engrossed in social networks. This is a widespread addiction hitherto unknown in the world and it is important to counteract it.

I include Walnut Remedy in most of the formulas I prepare in order to help children and adolescents to let go of habits and addictions that no longer serve them and to support transitions in their life, enabling them to successfully shift to a state of mental and physical health and independence.

Taking the Remedy

Taking the Walnut Remedy gives a child or adolescent the protection they need during life changes, helps them to let go of behavior patterns, calms them during transitions and encourages them to follow their ambitions and fulfill their dreams and ideals.

A personal experience

Ben had trouble moving from his beloved kindergarten to first grade at school. He missed his kindergarten teacher and his friends who remained there. To him, the classroom seemed too big and he was afraid to go in. He felt he couldn't connect with the children in his class and the school seemed big, noisy and scary.

I prepared a bottle of Bach Flower Remedies for him with the following formula:

- **Walnut** – to improve his ability to move from one situation to another.
- **Rescue Remedy** – for calm and general balance.
- **Honeysuckle** – to soothe his longing for kindergarten.
- **Mimulus** – to address his fears of the large and noisy school.
- **Aspen** – to address his hidden fears.
- **Larch** – to strengthen his self-esteem.
- **Water Violet** – to improve his ability to connect with the children in his class.

Ben regularly received the Bach Flower drops every day as well as having them in his water bottle. After three days he was freer and calmer and after two and a half weeks he made friends with several children, happily entered the classroom, enjoyed participating in class, and stopped missing kindergarten.

34.
WATER VIOLET
Hottonia palustris

FOR LONELINESS AND SOCIAL DIFFICULTIES

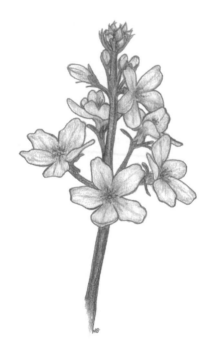

Water Violet Remedy is suitable for children and adolescents who trust only themselves, feel as if a glass partition separates them from those around them, spend a lot of time alone and tend to maintain a distance from others. These young people tend to be quiet and clever, to do everything alone and keep things to themselves. They are proud and independent and know how to keep themselves busy, learning and playing by themselves for long periods of time. They avoid arguments, are sad and solitary and are known for their ability to suffer sorrow and the deepest pain courageously and without telling anyone because they are reluctant to burden others. Because of their tendency to solitude and maintaining a distance from others, most children and adolescents they know tend to think of them as arrogant and superior.

Water Violet Remedy is suitable for supporting children and adolescents who are shunned or suffer from social isolation, who are on the autistic spectrum, or who have special needs.

The global Covid-19 epidemic imposed strict social isolation on us all for an extensive period of time and, consequently, many children and adolescents are more than ever in need of Water Violet Remedy.

Taking the Remedy

Taking Water Violet Remedy can encourage a child or adolescent to approach others and create relationships with their peers and with those around them, enjoying their company.

A personal experience

Twelve-year-old Lenny was an independent child who was talented and very clever, but had difficulty finding true friends. Most of the children in his class wanted to be with the 'king and queen' of the class and their group, frequently relating to Lenny with scorn because he was a good student and to them he appeared 'boastful and conceited'.

Lenny found it hard to create good relationships with other children and, since he wasn't invited to parties and social gatherings, he was socially isolated.

I talked to him and discovered an incredible child who was clever and mature for his age, who succeeded at his studies and hobbies but who, when he was with other people, felt he couldn't really get close to them, as if a glass partition separated him from others.

I prepared a bottle of Bach Flower Remedies for him with the following formula:

- **Water Violet** – to address his sense of loneliness and help him to connect with his peers in a calmer and better way.
- **Rescue Remedy** – for calm and general balance.
- **Walnut** – to improve his ability to move from a state of independence and loneliness to one of connection with his peers and people around him.
- **Mimulus** – to address his fear of making connections with others.
- **Aspen** – to address his hidden fears.
- **Larch** – to strengthen his self-esteem.
- **White Chestnut** – to calm his constant thoughts.

Lenny's response took several months, during which his attitude to himself improved as well as his relations with those around him. Today, he has several true friends and he feels a profound intimacy with them and enjoys being in their company.

35.
WHITE CHESTNUT
Aesculus hippocastanum

FOR TROUBLESOME THOUGHTS AND INTERNAL
ARGUMENTS

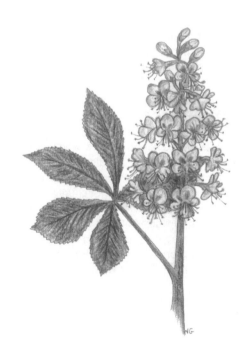

White Chestnut Remedy is suitable for helping children and adolescents who have difficulty calming their many thoughts, inner arguments and the unwanted ideas rushing about their mind. They tend not to listen to what is said to them, nor do they pay attention to their surroundings, and consequently they may get involved in accidents. Children and adolescents in need of White Chestnut Remedy suffer from stubborn, worrying thoughts and mental arguments; they often feel they cannot concentrate on their studies; and they'd give anything to calm the stream of thoughts rushing through their head.

White Chestnut Remedy can help children and adolescents who have difficulty falling asleep or who suffer from insomnia; it also helps them concentrate on their studies, particularly during exam time.

Taking the Remedy

Taking the White Chestnut Remedy can help children and adolescents 'empty their head', calm their thoughts, disconnect from problems and daily worries, focus on their studies and achieve clear and lucid thinking.

A personal experience

Nine-year-old Dina was an excellent student who worked hard at her studies, striving to excel at everything she did. Special exams were to be held at her school after which the children who succeeded would qualify for important supplementary classes at a local university, and teachers advised her to study the required material and take the exams. She was very happy to be chosen and started studying hard. However, while preparing for the exams, she was very tense and had difficulty sleeping at night. Her worried parents brought her to me for help.

I prepared a bottle of Bach Flower Remedies for Dina with the following formula:

- **White Chestnut** – to calm her thoughts, improve her capacity for concentration, and help her to fall asleep at night.
- **Rescue Remedy** – for calm and general balance.
- **Walnut** – to improve her ability to move from one situation to another.
- **Mimulus** – to address her conscious fear of failure.

Aspen – to address her hidden fears.

Elm – to help and support her during times of tiredness and lack of belief in her ability to succeed.

Larch – to strengthen her self-esteem.

Dina used the bottle of Bach flower remedies I prepared for her and felt much calmer. She managed to fall asleep at night, learned well, received excellent grades in all exams and joined the supplementary program at the local university.

36.
WILD OAT
Bromus ramosus
FOR HELP IN FINDING ONE'S DIRECTION IN LIFE

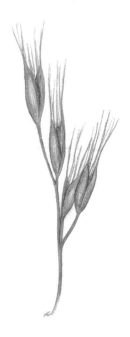

Wild Oat Remedy is suitable for helping ambitious children and adolescents who are successful, talented and strive to do something special in life and fulfill their potential, but who feel they haven't yet discovered their true calling. They tend to spread their energies among a number of areas of interest and various groups of friends; feel frustrated and dissatisfied due to unrealized ambitions and a lack of confidence in their future; and seek a suitable area or direction in order to find their calling and best fulfill their dreams and ambitions. They are faced with a choice of several directions in their life, and work hard to progress, but feel they can't get the best out of themselves and need a change and a significant goal that would give direction to their life.

Taking the Remedy

Taking Wild Oat Remedy can help a child or adolescent see their abilities clearly, choose the direction they want to take and discover the best way to manifest their ambitions.

A personal experience

Seventeen-year-old Aaron loved writing short stories, making animated drawings, singing and playing guitar, and he excelled in all areas in which he engaged. When the time came to choose a course of study and specialize in a particular field, he had difficulty deciding on his true life purpose and wasn't sure what he wanted to do in the long run.

I prepared a bottle of Bach Flower Remedies for him with the following formula:

- **Wild Oat** – to help him find his true calling.
- **Rescue Remedy** – for calm and general balance.
- **Walnut** – to improve his ability to move from one situation to another.
- **White Chestnut** – to balance the excess of internal argument in his mind.
- **Scleranthus** – to help him choose his preferred path.
- **Aspen** – to calm his hidden fears.
- **Larch** – to strengthen his confidence in himself and his abilities.

Aaron's parents told me that from the moment he began to take the Bach Flower Remedies, he calmed down and looked as if a burden had fallen from his shoulders. He told his parents: 'I used to think about all the things I loved doing and felt torn because I wasn't sure what I wanted to do. Now I realize that it's possible to combine several fields I love, to learn and specialize in them, manifesting my life's purpose. I simply feel that my purpose is calling me, and I know I will succeed!'

37.
WILD ROSE

Rosa canina

FOR A LACK OF INTEREST AND FEELINGS OF APATHY

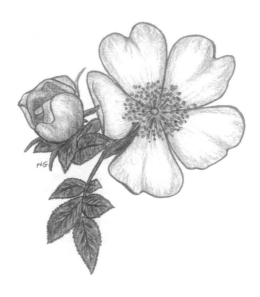

Wild Rose Remedy is suitable for helping children and adolescents who are completely passive, without motivation, joy or pleasure; they make no effort to feel better, but surrender to their fate, accepting the situation as it is, without expectation or motivation.

They tend to be bored and without energy, indifferent, apathetic, passive and somber; they avoid responding to what is happening around them, relating to life as a fixed fate they can neither oppose nor change.

This behavior is characteristic of adolescence when being 'cool' and showing no emotion are admired attributes, but that is supposed to be a passing phase. When their apathetic state becomes chronic, and they behave like this all the time, it is advisable to see a conventional specialist for advice.

Taking the Remedy

Taking the Wild Rose Remedy can help a child or adolescent find an interest, joy and meaning in life; it can improve their ability to act and respond, and it encourages them to shift from passivity to being proactive.

A personal experience

Sixteen-year-old Dean's friends called him 'Poker Face' because they'd never seen him get excited or respond in any way to the things happening around him. The teachers told his parents that he took no interest in his studies, and his parents were very worried because he didn't seem to be interested in any field and spent his days passively watching television or his mobile phone screen.

When talking to Dean, I realized that he was simply indifferent, had no desire to do anything and, to him, his life seemed boring and purposeless; he didn't believe something good or interesting could happen to him.

I prepared a bottle of Bach Flower Remedies for him with the following formula:

- **Wild Rose** – to improve his ability to take an interest in life.
- **Rescue Remedy** – for calm and general balance.
- **Walnut** – to improve his ability to move from one situation to another.

- **Larch** – to strenghten his self-confidence.
- **Wild Oat** – to encourage his ability to find a goal and a purpose in life.
- **Mimulus** – to address his fear of showing his feelings.

After a few days of taking the Bach Flower Remedies, Dean began to take an interest in what was happening around him. After about six months, I met his mother who told me that a great change had taken place in him. His studies had improved and he'd joined a scout movement. Today he takes great interest in many areas of life.

38.
WILLOW

Salix vitelline

FOR BITTERNESS AND THE TENDENCY TO ENVY OTHERS

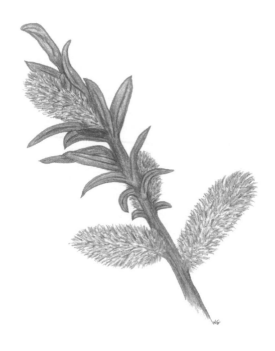

Willow Remedy is suitable for children and adolescents who are bitter and full of self-pity; these young people are somber, angry, embittered, resentful and love to argue. They compare themselves to others and tend to envy their happiness and good luck, always believing that the destiny of others is better than their own. When they are scolded or punished, they feel that there is no justice in the world, claiming that people are stricter with them than with other children.

Children in need of Willow tend to frown and complain and sometimes the reason for their distress isn't clear. They always blame others for their situation, are full of self-pity and 'eat their heart out'. They have difficulty accepting wrongdoing and blame the whole world for any obstacle, saying 'It isn't fair'. When they are given something, or are helped, they take it for granted, without acknowledging it because they are sure they deserve it.

Willow Remedy is also highly suitable for a child or adolescent experiencing temporary resentfulness.

Taking the Remedy

Taking Willow Remedy can help children and adolescents realize that they create their own reality by focusing on specific aspects of life, enabling them to stop feeling like victims and helping them to achieve mature and responsible emotional equilibrium and live in a happier and more optimistic way.

A personal experience

Five-year-old Rachel returned home and angrily told her mother about her day in kindergarten: 'Everyone got chocolate, but my square was the smallest... and the kindergarten teacher got mad at me because other children were making a noise... it's not fair... everyone was making a noise, but she only told me to 'sit quietly!' She used to complain that her dresses weren't as pretty as her friend Barbara's; she was resentful every time she felt deprived, and her family would call her 'Mrs Bitterbutter'.

I prepared a bottle of Bach Flower Remedies for Rachel with the following formula:

- **Willow** – to counteract her sense of bitterness and jealousy.
- **Rescue Remedy** – for calm and general balance.
- **Walnut** – to improve her ability to move easily from one situation to another.
- **Mimulus** – to address her conscious fears of discrimination and injustice.
- **Aspen** – to address her fears of the unknown.
- **Holly** – to address her jealousy of her friend.

Rachel's mother gave her the Bach Flower Remedies four times a day and added them to her personal water bottle.

After three weeks, her mother called me to say that 'Mrs Bitterbutter' had completely changed. Her constant complaining had diminished, she was full of joy, and life with her was much better and more pleasant.

RESCUE REMEDY

FOR HELP IN ANY EMERGENCY TO ACHIEVE CALM AND
GENERAL BALANCE

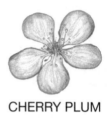

CHERRY PLUM

STAR OF BETHLEHEM

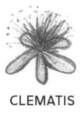

CLEMATIS

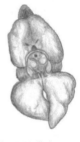

IMPATIENS

ROCK ROSE

The Rescue Remedy formula consists of a powerful combination of five different Bach Flower Remedies. The original formula was created by Dr Edward Bach in order to help with a wide variety of emergencies. Today, it is famous all over the world and is sold as part of the Bach Flower Remedy kit as well as in a separate bottle, intended to provide help with situations of difficulty, stress and anxiety.

The Rescue Remedy formula consists of:

- **Star of Bethlehem** – for relieving trauma, mental and physical shock and numbness.
- **Rock Rose** – to address terror and panic.
- **Impatiens** – to counteract emotional distress, nervousness and stress.
- **Cherry Plum** – to address violent outbursts and hysteria.
- **Clematis** – to help with situations of profound confusion, a sense of fogginess and/or loss of consciousness.

When preparing a personal formula for a child or adolescent, we can add the Rescue Remedy formula to the other Remedies we have chosen, as in the cases listed above.

In the course of the years I've been using and teaching about Bach Flower Remedies, I've realized that when Rescue Remedy is included in a young person's first personal formula, the results are excellent.

The Rescue Remedy formula in its original bottle is considered a Remedy in its own right, so we can choose up to another six further Remedies to accompany it when preparing a personal formula.

I include Rescue Remedy in most of the first personal formulas and decide later on whether or not to include it in follow-up formulas.

Choosing suitable Bach Flower Remedies

Choosing Bach Flower Remedies can be done primarily in two ways: by asking questions or by intuition. Anyone can choose the method best suited to them and can also combine the two methods. When meeting with a child or adolescent, I note down what I think are the most suitable Remedies and, in the course of the conversation, or at the end, I suggest they look at and sense which of the original Bach Flower bottles most 'attracts' them.

Choosing Bach Flower Remedies by asking questions

Choosing by asking questions takes place in conversation with the child or adolescent, as detailed on page 16, and/or in conversation with the parents or care-givers.

It is advisable to note down the main points of the conversation and the names of the Bach Flower Remedies you think are suitable for treating the issues that arise in the conversation, making sure that the combination of Remedies in the formula includes Type Remedies (page 138), Situation Remedies (page 139) and Support Remedies (page 140). Then, prepare the formula accordingly.

Energetic choice of Bach Flower Remedies

The energetic choice of the original Bach Flower Remedy bottle is based on the child or adolescent's reaction and senses. When a specific remedy is good for their body and mind, they will feel 'attracted' to it, wanting to pick it up and, when a specific remedy isn't right for them, they will sense this and be 'repelled' by it and won't want to touch it. Since most children and adolescents have never experienced energetic methods of choice, it's important to explain to them that this is a moment to pay attention to their body's intuitive responses and internal sensations. Ask the young person to tell you which original Bach Flower Remedy bottle 'attracts' them and what they feel about it.

There are many ways to choose energetically and each person can choose to do so in the way that best suits them.

Energetic methods of choosing Bach Flower Remedies

Observing the Remedies

In the course of the therapeutic session, I place the wooden box containing the original Bach Flower Remedies in the middle of my work table in the clinic and suggest to the child or adolescent they examine the original bottles the Remedies are supplied in and point to those that particularly attract them.

Many children are glad to cooperate and I've discovered that they are capable of intuitively choosing the Bach Flower Remedies that are appropriate for them.

Passing your hand over the Remedies

When I place the wooden box of Bach Flower Remedies on the table, many children and adolescents are drawn as if by magic to the original Remedy bottles, instinctively putting out a hand and asking if they can touch these. I ask anyone who asks this to pass their hand gently about 10-15 centimeters above each bottle without touching it. Then I ask them which bottle most 'attracts' them or feels most pleasing to them and to choose that one. It is wonderful to see how children and adolescents are attracted to and choose the Remedy best suited to them.

Choosing a Remedy with eyes closed

When a child or adolescent says it is difficult for them to choose, I suggest they close their eyes, pass their hand slowly about 10-15 centimeters above each original Remedy bottle without touching it and, when they feel their hand drawn gently downward, to open their eyes and point to the bottle that attracts them. Choosing with closed eyes best enables a child or adolescent to connect with their senses and most Remedies chosen in this way are the ones most suited to their needs.

Creating treatment formulas

The 38 Bach Flower Remedies help us create a unique treatment formula that is personally adapted for each child or adolescent.

Each personal formula contains one to seven Remedies selected according to the complete and in-depth diagnosis we have made. **Do not use more than seven remedies in a formula**.

For a comprehensive and active formula, it is advisable to combine three categories of Remedy: a Type Remedy, a Situation Remedy and a Support Remedy.

Type Remedies

Each Remedy in this book precisely captures a particular character trait that a child or adolescent might be manifesting. These traits are included in the descriptions of each Remedy. When a Remedy relates to a young person's **characteristic behavior** we call it a Type Remedy. We use Type Remedies for long-term treatment of problems related to a child or adolescent's typical traits, qualities and behaviors over time.

Situation Remedies

The behavior of children and adolescents is affected by everything going on in their daily life as well as by the behavior of those around them. When we see that their behavior has significantly changed, we have to take on board that they are currently facing a new situation, or experiencing a change in some area of their life, and that everything currently happening in their life is affecting them and how they behave. We must find out the real nature of their situation, what is currently happening and the root of their problems in order to understand how we can help them to become calm and balanced. When we read the description of a particular Remedy in this book and find that it matches the child or adolescent's **current behavior**, we can use it to address that. A Remedy chosen for this reason is therefore known as a *Situation Remedy*. We use a Situation Remedy for a specific, current and focused treatment of a child or adolescent for the period required.

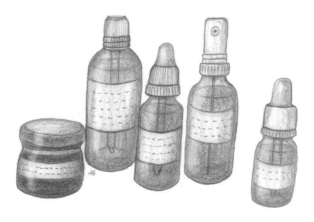

Support Remedies

Certain Bach Flower Remedies are suitable for support in various situations and can be included in personal formulas as required.

Walnut Remedy supports situations of transition, helping a child or adolescent to pass from one situation to another, successfully coping with all the changes and transitions in their life.

Larch Remedy supports children and adolescents', emotional resilience, reinforcing their self-confidence and helping them to believe in their abilities.

Olive Remedy supports a child or adolescent's body, helping them to cope with physical and mental tiredness, regain their strength and recover from their illness.

Scleranthus and Cerato Remedies (adapted personally for the child or adolescent) support situations of indecisiveness, helping them to make the best possible decision.

Aspen and Mimulus Remedies (adapted personally for the child or adolescent) provide help and support in situations of fear and anxiety.

Rescue Remedy supports any personal formula, enabling a child or adolescent to enjoy their own formula with a light dose of first aid remedies.

Preparing a Bach Flower Remedy formula bottle for children of all ages

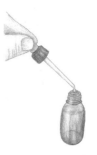

In order to prepare bottles for Bach Flower Remedy formulas, we can buy the original, individual Bach Flower Remedy bottles at many health food stores and pharmacies. It is possible to buy the whole kit, which contains all 38 Remedies plus Rescue Remedy, or individual Remedies as required.

Mineral water is recommended as the base for preparing Bach Flower formulas for children of all ages. Various studies have shown the wonderful energetic properties of water, and mineral water is the cleanest and best energetic base you can use. If you cannot get hold of mineral water, it is possible to use filtered water.

To prepare a personal formula, fill a designated glass bottle of 30 ml, 50 ml or 100 ml with mineral water up to the shoulder of the bottle, and add 4-6 drops of each selected Remedy. It is possible to combine up to seven Remedies in each formula.

It is advisable to store prepared bottle of combined Remediess in the fridge and to distance these from electrical appliances that emit radiation, such as mobile phones, microwave ovens and televisions.

Method of preparation

1. Select the appropriate Bach Flower Remedies as detailed in this book, and devise a formula that contains up to seven of them.

2. Add 4-6 drops from each chosen Bach Flower Remedy to the glass bottle of mineral water and close it tightly with a lid or dropper. It is customary to use bottles of 30 ml, but when a larger amount is required, it is possible to use a 50-ml or 100-ml glass bottle. Use the same number of drops of each Bach Flower Remedy (4-6) no matter the size of the bottle.

3. On a label prepared in advance, write the name of the child or adolescent for whom you have made the treatment formula, the date of preparation and the formula details, including the names of all the Remedies added and how to use it. Stick this onto the bottle.

4. Hold the neck of the bottle in your dominant hand and gently tap the bottom of the bottle on the center of your opposite palm 100 times in order to charge it with positive, healing energy. While tapping, it is advisable to silently wish the child or adolescent for whom you have prepared the formula health, success and joy. The energetic charging of the treatment bottle is performed only once, during its initial preparation.

5. In order to prepare a water bottle for the child or adolescent, we can charge their personal water bottle with the appropriate Bach Flower Remedies. It is possible to use a water bottle of any size that is comfortable for the child or adolescent to carry with them. Fill the personal water bottle with mineral or filtered water and add 6 drops from the child or adolescent's personal treatment bottle. Close the lid of the water bottle, hold it by the neck in your dominant hand and gently tap the bottom of the bottle on the center of your non-dominant palm 100 times. Again, it is advisable to silently wish the child or adolescent for whom you have prepared the bottle, health, success and joy. After energetically charging the bottle, the child or adolescent may unrestrictedly drink from the bottle whenever they wish. When their personal water bottle is empty, it is advisable to wash it thoroughly, and start the process again.

Using the Bach Flower Remedy formula bottle

The recommended dose for a child or adolescent is 4-6 drops from the prepared formula bottle four times daily:

- first dose when the baby, child or adolescent wakes in the morning.
- second dose towards noon.
- third dose in the afternoon.
- fourth dose before going to bed.

In addition, it is possible to take the formula whenever required, for example, in situations of stress, before exams, after trauma, etc. You can:

- add 4-6 drops of the prepared formula to a glass of water and give a fresh glass to the child to drink four times a day and/or as required.
- add 4-6 drops to the bath water of a child or adolescent.
- rub up to 6 drops into the skin of a child or adolescent.
- create a treatment spray (see page 144) or treatment cream (see page 145) and use this when required.

Preparing a Bach Flower Remedy spray

A Bach Flower Remedy spray is meant for quick use anywhere by spraying the appropriate external area of the body – for example, an itchy mosquito bite, or a painful knee.

You can prepare a Bach Flower Remedy spray in a 30-ml, 50-ml or 100-ml glass bottle closed with a spray top.

To prepare the spray, fill the chosen glass bottle to the shoulder with mineral water, add the chosen Bach Flower Remedies according to the formula decided upon, and prepare the spray bottle in exactly the same way as a Bach Flower Remedy treatment bottle is prepared.

Preparing a Bach Flower Remedy cream

Bach Flower Remedy creams contain the Bach Flower formula adapted for treating the child or adolescent, and are intended to be rubbed into the skin in order to help physical and mental recovery in various situations. The cream can be used, for example, to calm the skin after prolonged exposure to the sun, to ease stiff muscles or to calm various pains.

Treatment creams are prepared by adding the selected Bach Flower Remedies to a base, delicate cream, prepared only from natural materials, such as coconut oil, shea butter or aloe vera gel. Alternatively, buy a natural cream that suits your personal preference to use as the base cream.

It is essential to:
- **Make sure that the child or adolescent is not allergic to any component of the base cream.**
- **Do not rub Bach Flower Remedy creams into cuts, open sores, burns, etc.**

Prepare the following in advance:
1. A glass jar of the desired size, with a screw lid.
2. A wooden spoon or stick to transfer the cream into the jar and stir it.
3. A delicate base cream, made out of natural, unperfumed materials. It is possible to buy a suitable cream or prepare it yourself, as detailed below.

4.   The Bach Flower Remedies formula you have chosen according to the needs of the child or adolescent.
5.   The required Bach Flower Remedies to make up the formula.
6.   A label on which to write down the details of the cream.

Preparing the cream

1.   Put the cream base into the glass jar you have chosen.
2.   Choose the appropriate Remedies using one of the methods suggested above (page 136), and prepare a formula containing up to seven Remedies.
3.   Add 4-6 drops from each chosen Remedy to the cream in the glass jar.
4.   After adding all the Remedies to the cream, stir it clockwise in circles with a wooden implement 100 times. While stirring, it is recommended to silently wish the child or adolescent for whom you are preparing the cream health, success and joy.
5.   Tightly close the lid of the glass jar of cream that you have pre-pared. Hold the jar in your dominant hand and gently tap the bottom of it on the center of your non-dominant palm 100 times in order to charge the cream with positive, healing energy. While tapping, silently wish the child or adolescent for whom you are preparing the cream health, success and joy. The energetic charging of the treatment cream is performed only once, during its preparation.
6.   On a label prepared in advance, write the name of the child or adolescent for whom you have made the cream, the date of preparation and the formula details including the names of all the Remedies added to the cream and how to use it. Stick this onto the cream jar.

Natural bases for Bach Flower Remedy creams

It is possible to use coconut oil, shea butter or aloe vera gel as a base for preparing Bach Flower Remedy creams.

1. Organic coconut oil. Throughout history, coconut oil has been recognized as beneficial for skin and hair. When you wish to use coconut oil as a base cream, make sure you buy a high quality, organic, cold-pressed variety and keep it in the fridge to prevent it from becoming liquid on hot days. Put the desired amount of coconut oil into the glass jar you have chosen and prepare the treatment cream according to the instructions opposite. After preparing it, make sure to keep the jar of cream in the fridge so that the cream remains solid.

2. Organic shea butter. This is excellent for a variety of creams. Put the desired amount of shea butter into the glass jar you have chosen and prepare the cream according to the instructions opposite.

3. Aloe vera gel. Natural aloe vera gel is excellent for treating the skin. Put the desired amount of the gel into the glass jar you have chosen and prepare the treatment cream according to the instructions opposite.

General base formulas for treatment creams

Bach Flower Remedy creams are personally formulated creams containing a choice of the Remedies that is appropriate for addressing the problems of the individual child or adolescent.

Over the years, I have discovered formulas that enable the preparation of **general treatment creams** that are suitable for helping children and adolescents in a variety of situations. It is possible to prepare creams according to these general formulas and keep them in the fridge for use when required, or to use general formulas as a base for preparing personal formulas. To prepare general base formulas we use 4-6 drops of each Remedy noted in the formula and prepare the cream as instructed on page 146.

General base formula
- **Rescue Remedy** – for general calming treatment.
- **Crab Apple** – for general skin care and good absorption of the cream.
- **Walnut** – to reinforce the ability to move from one situation to a desired one.

Base formula for trauma
- **Rescue Remedy** – for general calming.
- **Star of Bethlehem** – for immediate treatment of trauma.
- **Walnut** – to reinforce the ability to emerge from a traumatic situation and shift from an existing situation to the desired one.
- **Crab Apple** – for general skin care and good absorption of the cream.

Base formula for skin care after prolonged exposure to the sun
- **Rescue Remedy** – for general calming.
- **Olive** – to strengthen the skin and improve its capacity for rehabilitation.
- **Walnut** – to reinforce the ability to move from an existing situation to the desired one.
- **Crab Apple** – for immediate skin care and good absorption of the cream.

We can use each base formula by itself or with the addition of 4-6 drops of each of the Bach Flower Remedies that we feel are most appropriate for the specific requirements of a child or adolescent. **We can include up to seven Bach Flower Remedies in each formula**. This means that, when choosing a base formula containing three Bach Flower Remedies, we can add one to four individually selected Remedies, and when selecting a base formula that contains four Bach Flower Remedies, we can add one to three additional Remedies.

The end... and a new beginning

The world we live in is constantly changing and these changes affect us and our children in every way. We want our children to be healthy and happy, but we are frequently helpless in the face of physical, mental and other issues that trouble them.

We inhabit a technological age in which many children and adolescents are disconnected from nature, eat industrially produced 'fast food' and watch screens for hours on end. They are affected by social networks and exposed to content that is unsuitable for their age.

Covid-19 has adversely affected children and adolescents as a result of isolation and lack of close physical contact with their peers, older family members and their community and environment. Because of the enormous disconnection we experienced as a result of the pandemic, it is more important than ever to connect with nature. Bach Flower Remedies enable us to help our children connect with the healing properties of nature and to feel better about themselves and their environment, creating a present and future world that will be better for all of us.

Good luck with the Remedies and I wish you abundant health and joy in your life!

May all of earth's creatures live healthy and happy lives!

Index

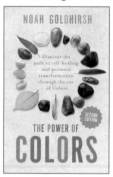
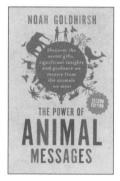